DRGGroupers Software & Services

A Catalog, Manual and Reference

By **Brendan F. Hemingway**
Lead Developer, DRGGroupers

REVISED October, 2009 (v27)

Library of Congress Control Number: applied for

ISBN 0-9819852-0-3

Printed in the United States of America

Cow and Calf Publishing
5 Spring Road
Branford, CT 06405

This publication is designed to provide information in regard to the subject matter covered. It is sold with the understanding that the publisher and the author are not engaged to render legal, accounting or other professional services. If legal advice or other expert assistance is required, the services of a competant professional should be sought.

Table of Contents

Introduction

This book is provided by DRGGroupers.com as a service to our customers. It is intended to help our customers in any or all of three different ways:

1. as a catalog of our software and services
2. as a manual of how to use our software or services
3. as an introductory reference to DRGs

This book is not intended as a general reference for Diagnosis Related Groups (DRGs). For general information about DRGs we refer you to Wikipedia's DRG entry,

`en.wikipedia.org/wiki/Diagnosis_Related_Group`

and to our own on-line Frequently Asked Questions (FAQ) page for DRGs,

`www.drggroupers.com/drgs.html`

However, we often are asked general questions about DRGs and different kinds of DRGs, so we provide our basic answers here to guide prospective customers (and avoid having to answer these questions on the phone or in email!)

DRG Basics

A DRG classifies an inpatient hospital stay on the basis of diagnoses, procedures, age, gender and discharge status into one of 500 mutually exclusive groups, numbered 0 to about 500.

There are two special DRG values: 0 (which means "not grouped") and 470 (which means "ungroupable"). The rest of the DRG values have descriptions, weights, LOS outlier trim points and mean LOS all of which depend on the DRG version.

DRG Historical Note

The original DRGs were invented at Yale University's Health Systems Management Group (HSMG) in the late 1970s. The principal researchers were John Thompson, a nursing guru, and Bob Fetter, an Operations Research kind of guy. Ron Mills, co-founder of the parent of DRGGroupers.com, was the technical lead and he was the one who created the biostatistical analysis package, AUTOGRP, which made the underlying research possible in real-time.

DRGs were adopted by the United States federal government's Health Care Finance Administration (HCFA) and first released in 1982 as version 2 (version 1 was the unreleased version which HCFA evaluated). Every year, on October 1st, HCFA releases a new CMS DRG version.

In 2001, the United States federal government's Health Care Finance Administration ("HCFA") became "the Centers for Medicare & Medicaid Services" or "CMS".

DRGs are good for providing a context in which to analyze hospital stays. DRGs were designed to allow hospitals to operate on a more industrial basis, with resource allocation and cost-center analysis, all of which were very hip in the late 1970s when DRGs were created. In a nutshell, DRGs predict likely resource consumption for any given hospital stay, allowing one to determine if the given hospital stay was too short, too long or just right.

Reimbursement

Originally, DRGs were designed to predict Length of Stay and were not concerned with reimbursement. However, following a study of their effectiveness as predictors of overall hospital resources required to treat different kinds of patients, DRGs were chosen by Medicare as the basis of the Prospect Payment System for hospitals. Since DRGs hit the scene as part of a reimbursement scheme, DRGs became linked with reimbursement in many people's minds.

Since DRGs measure resource consumption in the form of a normalized weight, using DRGs for reimbursement not only makes sense, it is easy: you multiply the DRG-specific weight by the facility-specific factor and voila! you have a reimbursement amount for a given inpatient stay. However, this additional step is called "pricing" and is not part of the grouper per se; it is a separate process which is not part of grouping. Software which makes this calculation is called a "pricer." For convenience, most pricer providers bundle the DRG grouper in with their software, which had confused grouping and pricing in many people's minds.

We are hardly experts on buying pricing software, but if you are looking to buy it and are stuck, check out 3M™ Health Information Systems. They seem to have lots of pricers out there in the world, so someone is buying them.

Federal DRGs

In the United States of America, the "official" definition of DRGs is the one defined by CMS (formerly HCFA). Strictly speaking, the CMS grouping algorithm is public, and anyone can implement it in software. (There are books published so that one could even do without the software and assign DRGs by hand.) However, CMS has blessed NTIS as the distributor of the reference grouper, which is written in IBM 360 Mainframe assembler. If you have an IBM 360-compatible computer, you can buy that grouper through NTIS and run that.

Other DRG Definitions

While we usually mean "US Federal DRGs" when we say "DRGs," there are many different governments which have defined their own version of DRGs. New York state defined their own. New Jersey defined their own for a while. France has their own, as does Portugal. Australia recently joined the club with their own version.

There are so many different DRG definitions because the federal DRGs are a bit of a compromise: The creators of the federal DRGs were constrained by the number of data elements that they could reasonably expect any given hospital in the country to collect. Furthermore, their baseline population is all Medicare patients, which skews the results somewhat.

As a result, the CMS DRGs are unambitious with respect to severity of illness and resource consumption and not appropriate to all hospital populations.

Many groups have tried to extend the basic DRG concept to fix these flaws. 3M™/HIS sells AP-DRGs ("All Payor" DRGs). Yale University's School of Medicine came up with RDRGs ("Refined" DRGs). CMS itself is working on SDRGs ("Severity-adjusted" DRGs).

Since DRGGroupers.com is constantly asked about RDRGs®, we asked the nice folks at HSC to give us a blurb to put on our website to answer this question. Here is their reply:

The RDRG severity-of-illness software is a product of Health Systems Consultants, Inc. in New Haven, Connecticut. The software groups inpatient hospital discharge data into DRGs and into severity classes within DRGs. The DRGs produced are identical to those of the public domain DRG grouper from the Health Care Financing Administration (HCFA--now CMS). The software assigns patients to 511 DRGs and to 1198 Refinement Group (RGN) numbers and is updated each year to conform to the CMS DRGs. Since the software system can predict hospital resource use, it can be used to improve hospital casemix analysis, analyze hospital performance, evaluate physician performance, measure quality, develop budgets, and to reimburse hospitals.

The RDRG severity-of-illness software was developed from a Yale University study funded by CMS (formerly HCFA) entitled, "DRG Refinement with Diagnostic Specific Comorbidities and Complications: A Synthesis of Current Approaches to Patient Classification." The study, completed in 1989, was designed to adjust the DRG system for the severity of a patient's illness. For information about the RDRG software, please contact Karen Schneider at

`karen.Schneider@healthsyst.com`

or call Health Systems Consultants at (203) 785-0650.

Diagnosis & Procedure Codes

The official federal grouper only accepts ICD9cm codes (International Committee on Diseases, version 9, Clinical Modifications) for both diagnoses and procedures. However, the American Medical Association has defined an alternative scheme for coding procedures, which they call CPT (Current Procedural Terminology). Many providers have chosen to code even in-house procedures using CPT. But if you want to group with CPT codes as input, then you have to convert them to ICD9cm codes first. This conversion is not a simple one-to-one mapping. Many vendors sell CPT-to-ICD9cm "crosswalks," but DRGGroupers.com is not one of them.

Assigning DRGs

The next chapter in this book will focus on DRG assignment software, so we will give only a cursory treatment here.

A DRG Grouper is a computer program or module which takes those 5 clinical and demographic data as input and gives a corresponding Diagnosis Related Group as output. The diagnoses and procedures are encoded as ICD9cm codes (International Committee on Diseases, version 9, Clinical Modifications). The age is a small integer from 0 to 129. The gender is encoded as 1 for male, 2 for female and 3 for unknown (don't ask). The discharge status, also known as "discharge disposition," is usually encoded either using UHDDS or UB92 (both medical billing standards).

The standard CMS (formerly HCFA) grouper, ours included, will accept up to 10 diagnoses, the first of which is presumed to be the Primary diagnosis. Likewise, up to 15 procedures are accepted, but their significance is determined by the grouping process, so their order is not important.

The relevance of any diagnosis or procedure code is determined by its attributes, which attributes are implemented as a "bit mask" or "mask" or "bit string." (You may see any of these terms in our documentation.)

The attributes guide the grouper in its use of any given code; for instance, the attributes say whether or not a code is gender-specific, or if it is allowed as a primary diagnosis. In addition to the information encoded in the attributes, the grouper applies logic to actually classify any given inpatient stay into a single DRG.

DRG Properties

Every DRG has certain properties. Those properties are:

- A DRG description (70 characters wide, version-dependant)
- An MDC (see the glossary for details)
- A Geometric Mean Length of Stay (GMLOS)
- A Weight (a normalized prediction of resource consumption)
- A Category: either "Surgical" or "Medical"
- A low "trim point" (the LOS below which lie the low outliers)
- A high "trim point" (the LOS above which lie the high outliers)

The DRGGroupers.com grouper returns all these and more: a set of flags for each of the Diagnosis Codes and Procedure Codes so that the caller can determine which codes were actually significant to the grouping.

New in 2008: POA, HAC

As of October 1st, 2008, there are two new concepts in DRG Assignment:

- A diagnosis attribute of "Present on Admission" (POA)
- Hospital Acquired Complications (HAC)

POA

The federal goverment is trying to get away from paying for medical mistakes; a common analogy is not paying a mechanic for a new car window if that mechanic accidentily breaks that window while fixing your brakes.

In order to avoid paying for medical mistakes, diagnoses are now flagged as having been present on admission (POA).

The values for the POA flag are not, as one might expect, simply Y or N; rather the following options are defined:

- Y for Yes -N for No -U for Unspecified -W for clinically undetermined -1 for unreported / not used / exempt from reporting

HAC

The logic which embodies handling the POA conditions is called the Hospital Acquired Complications ruleset. Some hospitals are exempt from the HAC, so the DRG assigment software has to be able to accept a flag which indicates that the institution from which these data come is exempt.

How To Use This Book

We expect that, in the usual case, the reader will start with this introductory section and then go to the chapter on the specific product about which the reader wishes to know more.

Note that the chapters often contain supporting information such as sample code for calling program modules or screen shots of interactive products.

However, we understand that the specific chapter may contain unfamiliar jargon, so we provide the glossary at the end of the book. We also understand that the specific chapter may contain unfamiliar concepts, so we provide a few explanatory chapters which immediately follow this introduction.

Syntax Notation

When giving the syntax of commands, we try to follow the standard notation. To us this means that optional arguments are written within square brackets, [like this], and required arguments are written within curly braces, {like this}.

```
command-name [optional] {required}
```

Lists of possibilities are given within vertical bars, like so:

```
[a|b|c]
```

which means "a or b or c";

Iteration is denoted by elipses, like so:

```
command-name {mode} [file...[file]]
```

which means "the command is called 'command-name', the mode argument is required and you don't have to give a file argument and you can give more than one file argument".

Link to M+H Consulting

DRG Groupers is a business unit of M+H Consulting. M+H Consulting is a medical information systems company who created DRG-related software to help them deliver service to their clients. A number of clients wanted to buy the software without needing any services, so M+H created DRGGroupers as a way of staying focused on their primary market. M+H continues provide software and technical support to DRG Groupers.

For more information on M+H Consulting, see their web site:

```
www.mhconsulting.com
```

DRG Assignment Software

Software to assign DRGs is also called a "DRG Grouper" or just a "grouper" for short.

If you are looking for general information about DRGs, please refer to the previous chapter in general and the section "DRG Basics" in particular.

If the jargon used here is unfamiliar to you, perhaps you will find definitions in the brief glossary of terms at the end of this book.

POA, HAC and Exempt Status

As of version 26, which was released in October of 2008, the notions of Present on Admission and exempt-from-Hospital-Acquired-Complications were introduced into DRG assigment. Our software supports these ideas if desired, and can ignore them as well, if required.

How Groupers Work

Like any other piece of software, groupers can be described with the Input / Process / Output model.

Input

There are five different parameters to a grouper which are needed for every Electronic Medical Record (EMR) to which a DRG is to be assign. Those parameters are:

• Patient age on admission, expected to be between 0 and 124

• Patient sex, coded: 1=male, 2=female

• Discharge status coded in either the UB92 standard or the UHDDS standard

- A list of up to ten ICD9cm diagnosis codes, in order of significance
- A list of up to fifteen ICD9cm procedure codes, in order of significance (and sometimes called "surgery codes")

In order to assign a DRG, a grouper needs access to a list of bit masks for every possible ICD9cm code. This list is called "the masks file" and is DRG version-specific.

Presenting ICD9cm Codes

Our software expects ICD9cm codes (either Diagnosis or Procedure) to be left-justified.

ICD9cm codes are officially of the form

```
code.subcode
```

but people often leave out the period. Our software accepts either convention.

Procedure codes are a maximum of four characters long (not counting the period) and Diagnosis codes are a maximum of five characters long (not counting the period). Our software optionally accepts Procedure codes with a leading 'S' to pad them out to five characters, if that is convenient. Trailing blanks are ignored.

However, LEADING blanks are a problem because they confuse the code handling subsystem: the subsystem assumes that the codes are left-justified and therefore that codes will leading blanks are entirely blank and to be ignored.

Please be sure to remove leading blanks on codes.

Process

The grouper uses these inputs to determine a DRG by applying both a specific DRG version's logic and the masks. As part of the process, a Major Diagnostic Category (MDC) is determined as well.

Output

In theory, a grouper could simply spit out a DRG for every input record. In practice, ther are a number of other, related, data elements that the user finds useful:

- A return code, indicating success or failure of the grouping attempt
- The MDC
- The DRG
- The Classification of the DRG
- A bit string of which Diagnosis codes were significant
- A bit string of which Procedure codes were significant

Return Codes

A return code of zero means that nothing went wrong. Any other value denotes a specific problem. For a list of the return codes for any DRGGroupers.com product, please refer to Appendix B.

Our Product Line

DRGGrouper.com's groupers come in a variety of forms. Figuring out which one you need can be difficult. To make this task easier, we have a wizard on our web site which will guide you through our product line:

```
www.drggroupers.com/cgi-bin/drgwiz.cgi
```

Supported Platforms

If our on-line wizard was not enough and our basic catalog did not answer your questions, the rest of this chapter is provided as a resource.

Our groupers are either for the UNIX platform or the Windows platform. Each of these platforms breaks down into specific versions, but we support a very long list of UNIX variants and all the major Windows versions.

We use an outside porting lab named Ready to Run to provide us with UNIX platforms on which to develop and test, so for an up-to-date list of UNIX variants that we support, please see their web site:

```
www.rtr.com
```

Our groupers are either stand-alone or embeddable. As a rule of thumb, end-users buy stand-alone groupers and programmers buy embeddable groupers.

Our stand-alone groupers are either batch-oriented or interactive.

This question does not arise for embeddable groupers because they can be embedded in either batch or interactive software.

ICD9cm Labelling

In addition to groupers, we sell a "helper" function which matches up an ICD9cm code with its short description. We did this because our customers really wanted the option of labelling each ICD9cm code with its description, especially in an interactive context.

This function is fast enough to be called on a character-by-character basis in a Windows application, providing a description for what the user has typed so far.

Stand-alone

"Stand-alone" groupers are independant, runable software applications. Stand-alone groupers are for end-users who want to assign DRGs to data.

Batch vs Interactive

Stand-alone groupers are further divided into batch groupers and interactive groupers. Batch groupers process a stream of input without human intervention. Interactive groupers prompt the user for input and return the corresponding DRG for that input.

Batch groupers are used to assign DRGs to a data set. Interactive groupers are used to give a human being a DRG for a given set of inputs.

Batch groupers are usually bought for use by system administrators or database administrators. Interactive groupers are usually bought for use by analysts or nurses.

Batch Groupers

The following is a list of our batch grouper products.

DRGFilt

DRGFilt is a console application grouper. DRGFilt runs under many varieties of UNIX as well in a DOS window on a PC. DRGFilt operates on text files. Usually you export your data to text, run it through DRGFilt and then import the results.

Excel-DRG

Excel-DRG is a Microsoft Excel spreadsheet which calls our Grouper DLL to assign DRGs to its rows. Included in the Excel-DRG purchase price is

1. Excel macro to call DLL
2. sample Excel spreadsheet with macro
3. Current Grouper DLL
4. DRG Masks file of your choice

A typical use of Excel-DRG is to assign DRGs to exported data. Almost any database management system (DBMS) can export data as text and import text as data. So the analyst usually does the following:

1. get the data to be grouped as a comma separated value file (CSV). Let us call this file "the original CSV."

2. load the original CSV into Excel-DRG's spreadsheet

3. cycle through assiging DRGs to the spreadsheet with the macro, perhaps changing the DRG version or cleaning up the data by looking for non-zero return codes and then assigning DRGs again

4. once the analysis is complete, the analyst often sends back the results by saving the Excel-DRG spreadsheet as a new CSV.

Interactive Groupers

The following is a list of our interactive grouper products.

Access-DRG

Access-DRG is a Microsoft Access application which collects the data needed to assign a DRG and stores that data, to be grouped by our Grouper DLL on demand. Access-DRG features interactive labelling of ICD9cm codes via our ICD9cm labelling DLL.

Included in the Access-DRG purchase price is

1. Access-DRG application
2. Current Grouper DLL
3. one DRG Masks file of your choice
4. ICD9cm DLL
5. ICD9cm Labels data file

CGI-DRG

CGI-DRG stands for "Common Gateway Interface DRG Grouper." CGI is the standard most webservers use to communicate with scripts.

CGI-DRG is intended to be installed by your IT department on an internal server.

CGI-DRG provides a simple HTML form into which any user with a browser and web access to your server can fill in and get back a DRG, as well as indications of which codes were used in the grouping and the DRG's description, MDC, weight and mean.

We have tested CGI-DRG under GNU-Linux and Apache, so we expect our ANSI C source to compile and run under just about any UN*X and just about any web server. We have tested CGI-DRG under NT 4.0 and Windows 2000 running IIS.

*** NOTE: this product does NOT store its results

VB-DRG

VB-DRG is our Visual BASIC DRG Grouper and is intended for Windows desktop endusers who want to group records interactively without saving the results. Common scenarios include care co-ordinators spot-checking a medical record.

VB-DRG is a Visual BASIC form which collects the data needed to assign a DRG and then calls our Grouper DLL with that data. VB-DRG then displays the results on the screen (but does not save them anywhere).

VB-DRG features interactive labelling of ICD9cm codes via our ICD9cm labelling DLL. VB-DRG can support multiple DRG versions.

VB-DRG automatically detects the presence of any and all masks files and then presents the user with a list of versions supported by your particular installation.

If you want to keep your VB-DRG application current, you will need to upgrade every year by buying a new Grouper DLL (the price of which includes a new masks file). You will also need a new ICD9cm Labels data file to keep up to date.

Included in the VB-DRG purchase price is

1. VB-DRG application
2. Current Grouper DLL
3. DRG Masks file of your choice
4. ICD9cm DLL
5. ICD9cm Labels data file

*** NOTE: this product does NOT store its results

SA-DRG

SA-DRG is intended for users with a full screen at their disposal. If you are in a full-screen environment, such as a DOS prompt on a desktop Windows machine, or telnet to a UNIX server, and you want a group which can support up to 3 different versions at once and provide descriptions for your ICD9cm codes, then you want SA-DRG which stands for Standalone Grouper.

*** NOTE: this product does NOT store its results

Embeddable

"Embeddable" groupers are meant to be incorporated in other software applications. Embeddable groupers are meant for programmers who want to add DRG assignment capability to other software.

Different Kinds of Embedding

Programs consist of chunks of machine instructions which are linked together into an executable image. For our purposes, linking is the process of matching variable names with memory locations and function names with both a prototype (how to call the function) and a return value (how to get a result from the function). Linking allows "resolving" of names at run-time.

Static Linking

C Object under DOS or UNIX

Compiled computer languages, such as C, have a separate and distinct compilation phase and linking phase. Linking this way is called "static linking." Since there is a separate linking phase, one can embed our grouper in a C program at the static linking phase if one buys our C object file grouper.

However, this is only a viable option if the following conditions are met:

- you build your C program from source and can relink and redistribute it;
- you develop on a platform for which we can compile a C object file.

Dynamic Linking

DLL under Windows, SO under UNIX

Since so many developers do not want to rebuild their programs in order to add functionality, the concept of "dynamic linking" was born.

In dynamic linking, you compile a hook into your program and this hook knows how to resolve names at run-time: it searches a given path for object libraries for the specified name and then loads the object from the library as needed.

Under Windows, this functionality is provided by Dynamic Link Libraries, or DLLs. Virtually all common development environments for Windows support dynamic linking. Virtually all common desktop applications for Windows can call out to DLLs. Thus our grouper DLL can be called by Visual BASIC apps (such as our own VB-DRG) or by Microsoft Office apps, such as MS-Access or MS-Excel.

Under UNIX, this functionality is provided by Shared Objects, or SOs. Thanks to SWIG (www.swig.org), an Open Source project for cross-language compatibility, our grouper is wrapped in a shared object which can be called by the Perl interpreter or the PHP interpreter. We intend to add Python to the list by the end of 2009.

Embeddable Groupers

The following is a list of our embeddable grouper products.

Note about DLLs

Sadly, C and BASIC have different function calling conventions. This means that a DLL compiled for C cannot be used by BASIC. Thus all our DLLs come in two flavors. Please be sure that you order the right one.

Grouper DLL

We have packaged our grouper module into two DLLs: one uses Pascal calling conventions (as does Visual BASIC) and the other one uses native C calling conventions.

Choose the VB-Callable DLL (mhdrgvb.dll) to run with Access and Visual BASIC applications.

Choose the C-Callable DLL (mhdrg.dll) to run with applications created with Visual C++ (or some other Win32 C compiler).

ICD9CM Name DLL

We have packaged our ICD9cm description module into two DLLs: one uses Pascal calling conventions (as does Visual BASIC) and the other one uses native C calling conventions.

Choose mhicdvb.dll to run with Access and Visual BASIC applications.

Choose mhicd.dll to run with C, C++ or C# applications.

UNIX Embeddable Grouper API

All of our UNIX progam-callable groupers share a single Application Program Interface (API). For Perl and PHP, all the parameters are strings. For C and C++, the last two parameters are short integers. In all cases, all the outputs are strings.

The Inputs are as follows:

1. DRG version number

2. Path to the masks file or files

3. Discharge status

4. Patient age on admission

5. Patient sex (1=male, 2=female)

6. String of contiguous, left-justified, blank-padded ICD9cm DX codes

7. String of contiguous, left-justified, blank-padded ICD9cm Surgery (aka Procedure) codes

8. Length of each ICD9cm DX code

9. Length of each ICD9cm Surgery (aka Procedure) code

The Outputs are as follows:

1. Grouper Return Code (what error, if any, arose during grouping)

2. Major Diagnostic Category of assigned DRG

3. DRG assigned to this patient encounter

4. DRG version number used to assign this DRG

5. The Weight of this DRG (a normalized prediction of resource consumption)

6. The Geometric Mean Length-of-stay for this DRG

7. PorM flag: P if this is a "procedure" or "surgery" DRG, M if a "medical" DRG

8. DRG Description: the official name of this DRG

Perl Shared Object

Through the magic of SWIG, a wrapper-generator, we are able to access our C-callable object through Perl on many platforms. You install the shared object in the appropriate location, you 'use' our mhdrg.pm package and voila! you can assign DRGs in a Perl script. Thanks to the DBI package for accessing databases and Perl's many powerful features for handling text or parsing binary data, our module makes assigning DRGs to records in databases or in export files rather easy.

PHP Shared Object

SWIG (see above) also allows us to create a PHP module which assigns DRGs so that you, in turn, can add DRG assignment to your PHP applications

C-Callable Object

Our grouper is an ANSI C program which can be compiled by almost any valid ANSI C compiler. We have compiled our grouper under every one of our supported platforms with little or no modification.

Complete Product List

This is our basic catalog, a straight listing of our products in alphabetical order. However, we direct you to our web site for the latest information:

```
www.drggroupers.com
```

32 bit C-callable shared object

- Product ID: COBJ32SO
- Associated Files: c32_libmhdrg.so, drgman.pdf

- Comes with a masks file.

32 bit Linux CGI DRG Assigner

- Product ID: LINUX32CGIDRG
- Associated Files: cgi-drg_32, drgman.pdf
- Comes with a masks file.

32 bit Linux DRGFilt

- Product ID: LINUXFILT32
- Associated Files: drgfilt_lnx_32, drgman.pdf
- Comes with a masks file.

32 bit Perl-callable shared object

- Product ID: PERL32SO
- Associated Files: perl32_mhdrg.so, drgman.pdf
- Comes with a masks file.

32 bit PHP-callable shared object

- Product ID: PHP32SO
- Associated Files: php32_mhdrg.so, drgman.pdf
- Comes with a masks file.

32 bit Windows CGI DRG Assigner

- Product ID: W32CGIDRG
- Associated Files: cgi-drg.exe, drgman.pdf
- Comes with a masks file.

64 bit C-callable shared object

- Product ID: COBJ64SO
- Associated Files: c64_libmhdrg.so, drgman.pdf
- Comes with a masks file.

64 bit Linux CGI DRG Assigner

- Product ID: LINUX64CGIDRG
- Associated Files: cgi-drg_64, drgman.pdf
- Comes with a masks file.

64 bit Linux DRGFilt

- Product ID: LINUXFILT64
- Associated Files: drgfilt_lnx_64, drgman.pdf
- Comes with a masks file.

64 bit PHP-callable shared object

- Product ID: PHP64SO
- Associated Files: php64_mhdrg.so, drgman.pdf

- Comes with a masks file.

DRG Assignment Jumbo Data set

- Product ID: DASJUMBO
- This is a DRG assignment service, not a software product.

DRG Assignment Large Data set

- Product ID: DASLARGE
- This is a DRG assignment service, not a software product.

DRG Assignment Medium Data set

- Product ID: DASMEDIUM
- This is a DRG assignment service, not a software product.

DRG Assignment Small Data set

- Product ID: DASSMALL
- This is a DRG assignment service, not a software product.

DRG Masks

- Product ID: MASKS

DRGFilt for 32 bit Windows

- Product ID: WINFILT
- Associated Files: drgfilt.exe, drgman.pdf

- Comes with a masks file.

DRGFilt for AIX

- Product ID: AIXFILT
- Associated Files: drgfilt.aix, drgman.pdf
- Comes with a masks file.

DRGFilt for Sun SPARC

- Product ID: SPARCFILT
- Associated Files: drgfilt.sparc, drgman.pdf
- Comes with a masks file.

ICD9 Name-finding C-callable DLL

- Product ID: CICD
- Associated Files: mhi9tabf26.exe, drgman.pdf

ICD9cm Name VB-callable DLL

- Product ID: VBICD
- Associated Files: mhicdvb.exe, drgman.pdf

ICD9cm short file

- Product ID: ICDTAB
- Associated Files: icd9.tab
- This is an ICD9-related production, not a DRG assignment product.

ICL Run-time Environment Upgrade

- Product ID: ICLUP
- Associated Files: ide
- Comes with a masks file.

MS-Access DRG Assigner

- Product ID: ACCESSDRG
- Associated Files: MHGrouper.mdb, drgman.pdf
- Comes with a masks file.

MS-Excel DRG Assigning spreadsheet

- Product ID: XLDRG
- Associated Files: mhdrgvb.xls, mhdrgvb.exe, DischargeDispositions.txt, readme-excel.txt, drgman.pdf
- Comes with a masks file.

Perl-callable shared object

- Product ID: PERL64SO
- Associated Files: perl64_mhdrg.so, drgman.pdf
- Comes with a masks file.

VB-callable grouper DLL

- Product ID: VBDLL
- Associated Files: mhdrgvb.exe, drgman.pdf

- Comes with a masks file.

Visual C-callable DLL

- Product ID: CDLL
- Associated Files: mhdrg.exe, drgman.pdf
- Comes with a masks file.

Windows desktop app to assign DRGs

- Product ID: VBDRG
- Associated Files: mhvbdrg.exe, drgman.pdf
- Comes with a masks file.

DRG Assignment Service

If you want DRGs assigned to some records and you don't want to buy, install and run the software yourself, then our DRG Assignment Service (DAS) might be just what you are looking for.

Many of our customers are medical information analysts who do not have an on-going need for DRG assignment. Instead, they have the occasional dataset which they would like run through a grouper.

For these customers, we started a service which we call our DRG Assignment Service (DAS).

What Is The DAS?

The DAS works like this: you send us your dataset with some information about the file format and the record format. With that information, our software can find the data elements used in assigning DRGs. We run your dataset through our grouper and return the results to you along with a DRG summary report which gives you an overview of your dataset's DRG profile: a frequency distribution of DRGs assigned and errors encountered.

Required Data Elements

1. Patient Sex, usually represented by 'F', 'M' and 'U'

2. Patient Age at admission, or Date of Birth and admission date, from which we can calculate age at admission

3. Patient discharge disposition; see the Glossary for details. (We can default to 'unknown' if your data does not include this element.)

4. Up to ten ICD9cm diagnosis codes, in order of importance

5. Up to fifteen ICD9cm procedure codes, in order of importance

Version Processing Options

As part of the standard DAS, we offer two processing options: either we will use any supported DRG version on all your records or we will use the discharge date (which must be included in your dataset) to determine which federal DRG version was in use at the time of discharge and then use that version. Other methodologies for determining what version to use are possible, but would fall under the category of custom set-up programming and would require a custom quote.

Turn-Around Time

We guarantee three business days, but we can often deliver same day turnaround time if data is transferred electronically in both directions. For on-line transfers, we prefer SCP but will use FTP or email as required.

How Do I Send My Data?

You can send your data to us in any of several common formats:

- Microsoft Access database, either Access 97 or Access 2000;
- ASCII or EBCDIC text file with one record per line (either variable-width fields with a separator or fixed-width fields are ok);
- SQL INSERT statements in a text file (either ASCII or EBCDIC);
- MySQL database dump.

What Do I Get Back?

As part of the standard DAS, we will return any combination of the following data elements as fields in the output dataset:

1. Grouper Return Code (what error, if any, arose during grouping);
2. DRG Version used to group the record;

3. DRG Number assigned the record;
4. Major Diagnostic Category (MDC) of the assigned DRG;
5. The resource consumption weight of the assigned DRG;
6. The official description of the assigned DRG.

What Do I Do Next?

That depends on which return option you specify. The return options are:

1. At the beginning of the output dataset;
2. At the end of the output dataset;
3. As contiguous fields starting at a given field number;
4. As separate records with the same ID as the grouped input record (assuming that the input record has an ID field and that you have told us which field to use as the ID).

If we send you the DRG as part of your dataset, then you load we send you ON TOP OF your existing data. This would be any of the first three options listed above.

If we send you a separate DRG dataset, the fourth option listed above, then you load that separate dataset into a new table and link your existing data to that table by means of the record identifier.

Pricing and Custom Orders

In order to keep things simple all the way around, we offer this service as a flat fee by number of records in the input. If you can provide your data in any of the supported input formats mentioned above, then you qualify for the flat fee schedule. You can find the latest fee schedule at

`www.drggroupers.com/bureau.html`

If you cannot provide your data in one of these formats, it is likely that we can still help you, but you would have to contact us for a custom price quote. You can find our up-to-date contact information on-line:

`www.drggroupers.com/contact.html`

DRGFilt

If you are looking to assign DRGs to a dataset in batch mode, then DRGFilt might be just what you are looking for.

DRGFilt is a UNIX-style "filter" because it is a console application which reads from standard input and writes to standard output and writes its error messages to standard error. Non-filters usually read from a file and write to file.

Please review the earlier chapter entitled "DRG Assignment Software" and pay special attention to the "Presenting ICD9cm Codes" section.

Comma Separated Value files (CSVs)

DRGFilt operates on fixed-width field, one record per line text files. Back in the day, this was the prevailing standard. Times have changed and now the usual format is variable-width, comma-separated fields presented as one record per line.

Generally, any spreadsheet application can read in one format and spit out the other, so converting between fixed-width files and CSVs is relatively easy. We recommend that CSVs intended for processing by DRGFilt be converted via this pathway:

- load the CSV into a spreadsheet application

- save the spreadsheet as a fixed-with field file

(It is even possible to mix the two conventions, because sticking commas into the fixed-width record is harmless and having trailing blanks in CSVs is harmless. But we now discourage this technique unless you are very comfortable with text file manipulation as botching the mixed format file leads to confusion.)

Staying Current

DRGFilt is self-contained, to make it easier to deploy and use. But this means that to stay current you have to buy a new one every year. However, because our groupers are all backwardly compatible, you will still be able to use any previous version of DRGs for which you have a masks file.

How to Use a Filter

There are two ways to use a filter: either as an application or a step in a chain of processes.

Example of a filter as a process:

% filter < in-file > out-file

In this example, the program "filter" is reading from a file called "in-file" and writing to a file called "out-file".

Example of a filter as a link in a chain of processes:

% prog1 arg1 | filter | prog2

In this example, the chain starts with a program called "prog1" which takes an argument, "arg1". The output of prog1 is passed as input to a program called "filter" and the output of the program called filter is passed as input to prog2.

A typical use of DRGFilt is to assign DRGs to exported data. Almost any database management system (DBMS) can export data as text and import text as data. So the database administrator (DBA) usually does the following:

1. export the data to be grouped as a comma separated value file (CSV). Let us call this file "the export CSV."

2. run the export CSV through DRGFilt, creating new file with the old data and the DRG in it. Let us call this file "the import CSV."

3. import the import CSV into the DBMS, either overwriting the data in the database or just importing the DRG by

matching on a key

Command Line Arguments

DRGFilt's calling syntax is as follows:

drgfilt [-0|-1] {version} {masksfile} {control-file} < input > output

Because DRGFilt is a filter, you can also call it in this way:

prog1 | drgfilt [-0|-1] {version} {masksfile} {control-file} | prog2

or

prog1 | drgfilt [-0|-1] {version} {masksfile} {control-file} > output

The first argument is an optional switch. The possible values are either "-0" or "-1". This switch controls how the off sets within the control file are processed. See "Control File" below.

The second argument is the DRG version to be used. Note that DRGFilt can only handle one version at a time. See the "DRG Version" entry in the glossary in chapter 1.

The third argument is the name of the masks file which corresponds to the version specified by the previous argument. See the Masks File entry in the glossary in chapter 1 for more information.

The fourth argument to DRGFilt is the name of the control file to use. For more information, see "Control File" below.

Control File

The control file is a map for DRGFilt. The control file contains variable definitions which tell DRGFilt how to read variables out of the input and how to write result into the output.

In order to group, DRGFilt needs the five inputs mentioned earlier: a contiguous string of diagnoses, a contiguous string of procedures, an age, a sex and a discharge status. Since DRGFilt is meant to operate on arbitrary input records, each input record has to be described so DRGFilt can find what it is looking for. The control file is that description.

The control file also tells DRGFilt where you want it to write the results of its grouping.

The control file is a simple ASCII text file with one variable description per line. The fields in the description are fixed-width and always in this order: keyword, offset length.

Leading whitespace is not allowed.

The first 4 characters of every line are the keyword. The fifth character is ignored and is usually a blank for readability. Keywords can come in any order you like.

The next 3 characters are the offset, which is also followed by a spacer character.

Finally, the next 2 characters are the length.

Note: this is the parsing length, not the data length. In other words, this is the length needed to pull the data out of the record, not the length that the grouper will use. In particular, ICD9cm procedure codes are always four characters long, assuming that the period has been removed. Some programmers who create output files used by DRGFilt do not know how long the ICD9cm procedure codes are, so they leave extra room, often making the codes seven or ten characters long. In order to pull out the codes from the records, DRGFilt needs to know how wide the output field is. But the width of the output field only affects parsing, not processing.

In particular, many people have been confused by our example, taken from the federal government's own example. The creators of the federal government's test data set often leave many extra characters at the end of ICD9cm procedure codes. DRGFilt needs to know that those useless characters are there, in order to parse the record. But the grouper does not pay attention to any more than the leading four characters.

So an entry in the control file looks like this:

kkkk ooo ll

Where the k's are where the keyword goes and the o's are where the offset goes and the l's are where the length goes.

Either the '/' character or the '#' character can be used as the comment character.

Now we can explain the -0 and -1 switches. "-0" means "the control file offsets are zero-based," which is the default. "-1" means "the control file offsets are one-based." Zero-based offsets are offsets which start at zero, so the first position in the record is 0. One-based offsets are offsets which start 1, so the first position in the record is 1.

Input Keywords

NOTE: keywords whose length is less than four are padded at the end with blanks until the padded length is four.

The keyword "sex " (note the trailing blank) specifies where to find Patient sex, coded 1=male, 2=female.

The keyword "age " specifies where to find Patient age, expected to be 0-124.

The keyword "dx " specifies where to find the start of the contiguous diagnosis string of up to ten ICD9cm diagnosis codes. (See the glossary in chapter 1 for more information on ICD9cm codes.)

The keyword "dxl " specifies where to find the length of each diagnosis code in the contiguous diagnosis string. For this keyword, the offset is ignored.

The keyword "surg" specifies where to find the start of the contiguous string of up to fifteen ICD9cm surgery (procedure) codes.

The keyword "sgl " specifies where to find the Length of each code in the contiguous procedure string. For this keyword, the offset is ignored.

The keyword "ds " specifies where to find Discharge Status, coded following UB92 conventions. See the glossary in chapter 1 for details.

The keyword "recl" specifies where to find the input record length. This optional keyward was introduced with DRGFilt f16. If you don't specify a record length with "recl" then DRGFilt assumes that its input is a text file and that each line of the text file is a record. If you do specify a record length, then DRGFilt reads its input in chunks as big you specified, ignoring end-of-line markers.

New in 2008

The keyword "poa " specifies where, in the diagnosis code, to find the POA flag. If the diagnosis code length (specified by dlx) is 8, it is typical to find the POA flag at offset 7, that is to say the last character of every code.

The keyword "exmp" specifies that the institution from which these data come is exempt from the HAC.

Note that if neither of these keywords is present, the software assumes that POA is irrelevant and that the source institution is to be treated as exempt from the HAC.

Output Keywords

The keyword "drg " specifies where in the output record to put the DRG.

The keyword "mdc " specifies where in the output record to put the MDC.

The keyword "rc " specifies where in the output record to put the Grouper return code.

The keyword "ver " specifies where in the output record to put the version of DRGs being assigned.

The keyword "dflg" is short for "diagnosis flags." (This concept used to be called "the bit string.")

It is possible that for any given input record some of the diagnosis codes will be ignored as irrelevant to the group into which the record ultimately falls. In order to report which diagnosis codes were used and which were not, our grouper keeps a list of flags, one per diagnosis, of upto 16 diagnoses. These flags are boolean, which means that they are either zero, meaning "this code was not relevant," or one, meaning "this code was relevant." If you use the dflg keyword, your output will have a string of ones and zeros in it which tell you, in order, which diagnosis codes were used and which were not.

The keyword "sflg" is short for "surgery flags" because, once upon a time, "surgery" and "procedure" were synonymous. See the section on "dflg" for an explanation of the code flag data type. If you use the sflg keyword, your output will have a string of ones and zeros in it which tell you, in order, which procedure codes were used and which were not.

The keyword "morp" is short for "M(edical) or P(rocedure)" and will spell out either "Medical" or "Procedure" for as many characters as are specified by the length. If you specify a length of one, then only 'M' or 'P' will be output. If you specify a length of three, then either 'Medical ' or 'Procedure' will be output.

Sample Control File

Here is the control file we use to run DRGFilt against the standard CMS (formerly HCFA) test data set:

```
# DRGFilt control file for federal testdb
# there are 3 columns: name, offset and length
# -------------------------- input fields
age  000 03
sex  003 01
ds   004 02
dxl  000 06
dx   006 60
sgl  000 07
surg 066 70
# -------------------------- output fields
drg  195 03
mdc  198 02
rc   200 01
#
#'dflg' stands for "DX Flags" and 'sflg' stands
# for "Surgery Flags". (In ancient times, we called
#"Procedures" "Surgeries").
```

```
#
# these are bit-strings by which we mean strings
# of 1's and 0's. Each element of the string
# corresponds to a code. So the fifth element of
# dflag corresponds to the fifth Dx code.
#
# If an element is 1, then the corresponding code was
# used in the DRG assignment. If 0, then not.
#
# dflg represents all the DX codes.
dflg  201 10
# sflg represents all the Procedure codes.
sflg  211 15
# M or P attribute of the DRG that was assigned.
# Actually, either "Medical" or "Procedure" will be
# spelled out, depending on how long you make the
# output length.
morp  226 01
```

Installation

To install DRGFilt, you put the DRGFilt executable in a directory in the users' search path (often /usr/local/bin), and you put the masks file(s) and control file(s) in a directory which is readable by the users (often /usr/local/drggrouper or /usr/share/drggrouper).

WARNING: Tragically, a historical accident means that a leading dot in a masks file or path name will confuse DRGFilt, so please don't use masks file names or path names that start with "."

Typical Scenario

How is DRGFilt ususally used? Here is the typical scenario:

1. A database administrator (DBA) changes the database schema to include a DRG for every record (and perhaps other DRGFilt outputs as well, often the return code and version).

2. The DBA exports a dataset from a database management system, creating the file which is input to DRGFilt. Let us

call this file "the export file."

3. An analyst creates or customizes a control file for DRGFilt which matches the format of the export file.

4. A programmer or power user runs the export file through DRGFilt which creates output, which we will call "the results file."

5. The DBA imports the results file, overwriting the contents of the database.

And, voila! every record now has a DRG assigned to it.

Excel-DRG

Excel-DRG is for end users who are comfortable using Microsoft Excel and whose data is either already in a spreadsheet or can be put into a spreadsheet.

If you are not comfortable using Excel or if you cannot easily get your data into and out of spreadsheets then Excel-DRG is not for you.

Note: as of version 26, released in 2008, the DRG version can have either a 'p' or an 'e' or both appeneded to it. If there is a trailing 'p', it is assumed that the last character of every diagnosis code is a POA flag. If the there is a trailing 'e', then the source institution is presumed to be exempt from the HAC. Thus "26p" specifies POA support, while "26" does not. "25p" does not make sense.

Requires the DLL and Masks

Excel-DRG depends on our DLL for Visual BASIC and our masks files, both of which are included in the initial purchase price.

Note that you will have to refer to the chapter on the Grouper DLL for information about return codes, inputs and outputs.

Staying Current

Because Excel-DRG calls our DLL to do the actual grouping, you can keep it up-to-date by buying a new DLL every year and leaving Excel-DRG alone.

Because our groupers are all backwardly compatible, you will still be able to use any previous version of DRGs for which you have a masks file.

Technical Details

Excel-DRG is a Microsoft® Excel spreadsheet and macro which calls our Grouper DLL on every row. The results of the DLL call populate columns in the spreadsheet.

Our grouper DLL has the same inputs and outputs as all our other groupers. For details about how our groupers work, see chapter 2, "DRG Assignment Software." In particular, there is a section on inputs to our grouper and its outputs.

Typically, the user makes a copy of the original spreadsheet and works with the copy for every grouping project. The user then pastes or imports her data into the copy, sets the version column and calls the macro.

Columns of the Spreadsheet

The following is a brief description of the various columns of the spreadsheet.

Column A: ID Number

This column exists to link this data to your original dataset. A better name would have been "primary key".

Column B: Age

Required grouper input. See Chapter two for details.

Column C: Sex

Required grouper input. See Chapter two for details.

Column D: Discharge Disposition

Required grouper input. See Chapter two for details.

Column E-N: Diagnoses

Up to ten diagnosis codes. Required grouper input. See Chapter two for details.

Column O-AC: Procedures

Up to fifteen procedure codes. Required grouper input. See Chapter two for details.

Column AD: DRG Version

Required grouper input. See Chapter two for details.

Column AE: DRG

Optional grouper output.

Column AF: DRG Description

Optional grouper output.

Column AG: Grouper Return Code

Optional grouper output.

Column AH: MDC

Optional grouper output.

Column AI: DRG Weight

Optional grouper output

Column AJ: GMLOS

GMLOS stands for "Geometric Mean Length of Stay" and is often abbreviated to just "LOS". Optional grouper output.

Detailed Instructions

Open your copy of mhdrgvb.xls. Rows 2-6 contain test data. Before deleting these rows and populating the spreadsheet with your own data, we recommend that you try to group the test records. To do this, hit Ctrl-Shift-D (for DRG). You should hear a beep and see a message that 5 records were grouped.

Next, you can delete these rows. DO NOT ADD COLUMNS, DELETE COLUMNS, OR MOVE COLUMNS! Next, populate the spreadsheet with your own data.

The first column is your unique record identifier. Columns B-AD contain the information required by the grouper. NOTE: in addition to age, sex, discharge status, diagnoses and procedures, you must tell the grouper which version to use (for example, "F23"). The version is in column AD.

Columns AE-AJ contain DRG properties that were assigned by the grouper.

Once you have copied your data into the spreadsheet, run the grouper by hitting Ctrl-Shift-D.

Installation

Excel-DRG is delivered as a zip file. In the zip file you will find:

1. mhdrgvb.exe (installer for the drg dll)
2. mhmasksf23.exe (installer for the masks file)

3. mhdrgvb.xls (Excel spreadsheet for records to be grouped)

4. DischargeDispositions.txt (list of discharge disposition codes)

5. readme.txt (installation instructions)

In order for the Excel grouper to work, you must install both the DLL and the masks file. Double-click on mhdrgvb.exe to install the DLL. Double-click on mhmasksf23.exe to install the masks file.

Once those are installed, you can populate the spreadsheet with discharge data and run the Grouper. We highly recommend that you copy mhdrgvb.xls and use the copy as your working spreadsheet.

Access-DRG

Access-DRG is an interactive grouper.

Access-DRG is for Microsoft® Access users who are comfortable using MS-Access and whose data is either already in an MS-Access database or can be put into an MS-Access database.

If you are not comfortable using MS-Access or if you cannot easily get your data into and out of MS-Access databases, then Access-DRG is not for you.

Note: as of version 26, released in 2008, the DRG version can have either a 'p' or an 'e' or both appeneded to it. If there is a trailing 'p', it is assumed that the last character of every diagnosis code is a POA flag. If the there is a trailing 'e', then the source institution is presumed to be exempt from the HAC. Thus "26p" specifies POA support, while "26" does not. "25p" does not make sense.

Requires the DLL and Masks

Access-DRG depends on our DLL for Visual BASIC and our masks files, both of which are included in the initial purchase price.

Staying Current

Because Access-DRG calls our DLL to do the actual grouping, you can keep it up-to-date by buying a new DLL every year and leaving Access-DRG alone.

Because our groupers are all backwardly compatible, you will still be able to use any previous version of DRGs for which you have a masks file.

Technical Details

Access-DRG is a Microsoft® Access database and VBA module which calls our Grouper DLL on every row. The results of the DLL call populate columns in the database.

Our grouper DLL has the same inputs and outputs as all our other groupers. For details about how our groupers work, see chapter 2, "DRG Assignment Software." In particular, there is a section on inputs to our grouper and its outputs.

Typical Usage

Typically, one populates the database in Access-DRG however one likes (text file importation, ODBC calls, etc) and then fills in the form and then pushes the button to assign DRGs to every row.

After the DRG assignment has taken place, the DRGs are available either for export or for dynamic access.

CGI-DRG

CGI-DRG is an interactive grouper.

CGI-DRG is for users who want to enter data elements into a web form and have those data elements grouped into a DRG. CGI-DRG cannot save the results it gives, though you can copy and paste from your browser.

CGI-DRG takes the usual inputs and gives the usual outputs. For details about how our groupers work, see chapter 2, "DRG Assignment Software." In particular, there is a section on inputs to our grouper and its outputs.

CGI-DRG is used by care co-ordinators and nurses and medical records codes who want to see what different coding scenarios yield.

Note: as of version 26, released in 2008, the DRG version can have either a 'p' or an 'e' or both appeneded to it. If there is a trailing 'p', it is assumed that the last character of every diagnosis code is a POA flag. If the there is a trailing 'e', then the source institution is presumed to be exempt from the HAC. Thus "26p" specifies POA support, while "26" does not. "25p" does not make sense.

Staying Current

CGI-DRG is self-contained, which makes it easier to install and configure. However, it also mean that to stay up-to-date you have to buy a new one every year.

Technical Details

CGI-DRG is a program which is meant to be called by a web server. CGI-DRG is an ANSIC C program which used the Common Gateway Interface to communicate with the calling web server.

CGI-DRG only takes one argument: the PATH_INFO variable is assumed to be a readable directory name in which CGI-DRG can find the masks files.

Distribution

CGI-DRG is distributed as an executable for either the Win32 platform or for various UNIX platforms.

Supported Platforms

In theory, CGI-DRG should run happily with any reasonble web server.

Under UNIX, CGI-DRG has been tested with various releases of the Apache web server.

Under Win32, CGI-DRG has been tested with Microsoft's IIS web server.

Screen Shot

```
                                M+H CGI CMS (HCFA) DRG Grouper (2.1:21)

   M+H CGI CMS (HCFA) DRG Grouper
     ________________________________________________________________

Version: [f21] Age: 34_ Sex: [Female] Discharge Status: [Home______]
            Diagnoses 1-5: V3000* _____ _____ _____ _____
           Diagnoses 6-10: _____ _____ _____ _____ _____ Assign DRG


           Procedures 1-5: _____ _____ _____ _____ _____ Clear Form

          Procedures 6-10: _____ _____ _____ _____ _____
         Procedures 11-15: _____ _____ _____ _____ _____
DRG: 391 NORMAL NEWBORN
MDC: 15M Weight: 0.1536 Mean LOS: 3.10 Version: f21
     ________________________________________________________________

   © 2002,2003 M+H Consulting LLC, all rights reserved
```

In order to work in as many environments as possible, CGI-DRG uses as few graphic elements as possible. In fact, it is possible to use it in an all-character environment, such as a UNIX command line.

The screen shot above is what the form looks like in a UNIX command window, under the character-based browser "lynx". Note that the version is f21, the age is 34, the sex is female, the discharge status is home, the diagnosis code list has only one element and that code is "V3000" and there are no procedures.

CGI-DRG returned a DRG of 391 (Normal Newborn) which is in MDC 15 (which MDC is a medical MDC) and the weight is 0.1536, and the GMLOS is 3.1 days. Note also that there is an asterick after the V3000 code, which marks that code as having been significant in the DRG assignment.

Title Information

If you look closely, you will see that the HTML title of the CGI-DRG form in our example looks like this:

```
M+H CGI CMS (HCFA) DRG Grouper (2.1:21)
```

The string of numbers at the end, inside the parentheses, is the version of both the CGI-DRG software and the grouper logic it contains. This version string is of the form

```
major-version.minor-version:grouper-version
```

So our example's version breaks down like this:

```
2.1:21 = CGI-DRG version 2.1, Grouper logic version f21
```

This means that our example CGI-DRG has logic support for any federal DRG version from 2 through 21, inclusive. Providing that the corresponding masks files are detected, this particular copy of CGI-DRG can assign DRGs within any of these versions.

Masks Detection

Note that CGI-DRG offers the user a drop-down list box of available DRG versions. This list is created dynamically by scanning the specified directory for masks files and only listing versions for which there are masks files found.

For a masks file to be found, it has to represent a version of DRGs for which CGI-DRG has logic support.

Since grouping requires both logic and masks, the presence of a masks file by itself is not enough: for a version to be supported, the logic compiled into CGI-DRG has to handle that version. Our groupers are all backwardly compatible, so if CGI-DRG has logic support for version X, it also has logic support for all versions which came before X.

Return Codes

CGI-DRG pass through the following return codes with the following descriptions: (note that "DRG file" should really read "masks file")

```
 0 No Error
 1 Bad principal diagnosis
 2 Bad prin dx for MDC
 3 Invalid age
 4 Invalid sex
 5 Invalid discharge status
 6 Unspecified DRG error
 7 Invalid prin diagnosis
 8 No DRG file this version
 9 DRG number too high
10 Error in DRG file
```

Discharge Statuses

```
Unknown      -> 0
Home         -> 1
Other Hosp   -> 2
SNF          -> 3
```

```
ICF           -> 4
Other Inst    -> 5
Home Care     -> 6
AMA           -> 7
Expired       -> 8 (then mapped to 20)
```

Installation

Installation of CGI-DRG on any supported platform is the same: put the appropriate executable file in the appropriate directory and then publish the appropriate URL. Remember to append the directory name to the URL so that CGI-DRG can find the masks files. Then put the masks file or files into that directory.

1. copy cgi-drg or CGI-DRG.EXE to the appropriate directory so that your web server can find and run it

2. copy the masks files to a directory which is readable by your web server

3. remember to append the directory name to the URL when you run CGI-DRG

Sample UNIX URL

```
server.yourdomain.org/cgi-bin/cgi-drg/usr/tmp/drgmasks
```

In this example, the server is named "server" and that server is found in the domain named "yourdomain.org". The directory from which CGI-DRG is run is called "cgi-bin" (as is standard) and the PATH_INFO is "/usr/tmp/drgmasks" because that is where this particular UNIX sys admin put them. (A rather odd choice, since "tmp" directories are usually only for temporary files.)

Sample Win32 URL

```
server.yourdomain.com/cgi-bin/cgi-drg.exe/d:/tmp
```

In this example, the server is named "server" and that server is found in the domain named "yourdomain.com". The directory from which CGI-DRG is run is called "cgi-bin" and the CGI-DRG executable is called CGI-DRG.EXE. The PATH_INFO is "/d:/tmp" because the windows sys admin put the masks in D:\TMP. (This is a rather odd choice, because "tmp" directories are usually only for temporary files.)

VB-DRG

VB-DRG is an interactive grouper.

VB-DRG is for users who want to enter data elements into a MS-Windows desktop application and have those data elements grouped into a DRG. VB-DRG cannot save the results it gives.

VB-DRG takes the usual inputs and gives the usual outputs. For details about how our groupers work, see chapter 2, "DRG Assignment Software." In particular, there is a section on inputs to our grouper and its outputs.

VB-DRG is used by care co-ordinators and nurses and medical records codes who want to see what different coding scenarios yield.

Note: as of version 26, released in 2008, the DRG version can have either a 'p' or an 'e' or both appeneded to it. If there is a trailing 'p', it is assumed that the last character of every diagnosis code is a POA flag. If the there is a trailing 'e', then the source institution is presumed to be exempt from the HAC. Thus "26p" specifies POA support, while "26" does not. "25p" does not make sense.

Requires the DLL and Masks

VB-DRG depends on our DLL for Visual BASIC and our masks files, both of which are included in the initial purchase price.

ICD9cm Labelling

VB-DRG labels ICD9cm codes as you type them, giving you both a description and a cross-check on your data entry.

Staying Current

Because VB-DRG calls our DLL to do the actual grouping, you can keep it up-to-date by buying a new DLL every year and leaving VB-DRG alone.

Because our groupers are all backwardly compatible, you will still be able to use any previous version of DRGs for which you have a masks file.

Technical Details

VB-DRG is a Visual BASIC application which runs on any Win32 platform.

Distribution

VB-DRG is distributed with an installer to allow you to install or uninstall it cleanly.

Title Information

If you look closely, you will see that the title of the VB-DRG window looks like a long string of stuff. It breaks down into two parts. First, there is the identifier for VB-DRG itself:

```
VB-DRG from M+H Consulting,LLC
```

This is followed by the version string of the DLL VB-DRG is calling:

```
mhdrg.dll v1.5 (c) 2002 M+H Consulting, LLC:f23
```

In this example, the DLL version is 1.5 and the logic it supports is the f23 DRG version and before.

Masks Detection

Note that VB-DRG offers the user a drop-down list box of available DRG versions. This list is created dynamically by scanning the registry for masks files and only listing versions for which there are masks files found.

For a masks file to be found, it has to represent a version of DRGs for which VB-DRG has logic support.

Since grouping requires both logic and masks, the presence of a masks file by itself is not enough: for a version to be supported, the logic supported by the current DLL has to handle that version. Our groupers are all backwardly compatible, so if there is logic support for version X, there is also logic support for all versions which came before X.

SA-DRG

SA-DRG is an interactive grouper.

SA-DRG stands for "Stand-Alone DRG Grouper." SA-DRG is for users who want to enter data elements into a DOS window or a UNIX prompt.

Since SA-DRG was created for medical records coders, it has a number of features not found in LAT-DRG or Mini-DRG:

1. ICD9cm labelling

2. Ability to handle up to three DRG version simulanteous

3. Ability to shuffle the order of the Diagnosis and Procedure codes in order to most accurately reflect the medical record

SA-DRG does not save its results.

Note: as of version 26, released in 2008, the DRG version can have either a 'p' or an 'e' or both appeneded to it. If there is a trailing 'p', it is assumed that the last character of every diagnosis code is a POA flag. If the there is a trailing 'e', then the source institution is presumed to be exempt from the HAC. Thus "26p" specifies POA support, while "26" does not. "25p" does not make sense.

Staying Current

SA-DRG is self-contained, which makes it easier to install and configure. However, it also mean that to stay up-to-date you have to buy a new one every year.

You get a new masks file with every purchase and SA-DRG is backwardly compatible, so if you buy version X one year and version Y the next, you will still be able to assign version X DRGs with the new SA-DRG.

Technical Details

SA-DRG is an ICL application which means it can be run under Win32 or various UNIX environments.

SA-DRG takes the usual inputs and gives the usual outputs. For details about how our groupers work, see chapter 2, "DRG Assignment Software." In particular, there is a section on inputs to our grouper and its outputs.

ICL

See the chapter on ICL for details.

Supported Platforms

SA-DRG runs under most UNIX variants, MS-DOS and Win32.

Installation

Since SA-DRG is a simple ICL app, the installation process is rather simple:

1. create a directory, such as 'SA-DRG' and go to that directory
2. copy the interpreter (ide or IDE.EXE) to that directory
3. copy the application library (sadrg.lib) to that directory
4. copy the masks file or files to that directory
5. run the program with the supplied .BAT file or directly

```
ide sadrg.lib {low-version}
```

Screen Shot

```
                         M+H Stand-alone HCFA DRG Grouper
Code  Diagnosis - Description  Grprs       Code Procedure - Description  Grprs
V3000 SGL LB,IN HOSP,WO CESARE 9:;       1-
                                         2-
                                         3-
                                         4-
                                         5-
                                         6-
                                         7-
                                         8-
                                         9-
  Age:  34                              10-
  Sex: Female                           11-
Dstat: Home                             12-
# Diags: [1]    # Procs: [ 0]           13-
VN DRG/MDC                              14-
19 391/15 NORMAL NEWBORN
            Weight: [ 0.1524]   Trim Point: [    0]   Mean LOS: [   3.10]
20 391/15 NORMAL NEWBORN
            Weight: [ 0.1517]   Trim Point: [    0]   Mean LOS: [   3.10]
21 391/15 NORMAL NEWBORN
            Weight: [ 0.1536]   Trim Point: [    0]   Mean LOS: [   3.10]
                     Quit    Insert    Edit    DxSwap   PrSwap
```

Data Entry

SA-DRG is a full-screen application, which means that the display stays fixed and the data changes in the set positions.

SA-DRG is not aware of the mouse.

SA-DRG will automatically go onto the next field when the current field fills up. You can move on to the next field by hitting the Tab key.

You can bring up drop-down menus by hitting the spacebar. You can navigate within the menus with the left and right arrow keys; the up and down arrow keys move off of the menu. You select the highlighted item by hitting Return (also known as the Enter key).

You can skip to the end of form by hitting the Escape key. In some environments, such as telnet, you have to hit the Escape key twice in rapid succession to send an Escape to the application.

You can navigate the menu at the bottom with the arrow keys or the inital letter of the item you wish to highlight. You select the highlighted item by hitting return.

The menu items are as follows:

Quit means "I want to stop using SA-DRG"

Insert means "clear the form and start a new grouping"

Edit means "let me change this grouping"

DxSwap means "let me change the ranking of a diagnosis code"

PrSwap means "let me change the ranking of a procedure code"

Results

SA-DRG gives the standard results in the section at the bottom of the display, one set of results for each of the versions:

```
VN DRG/MDC
19 391/15 NORMAL NEWBORN
          Weight: [ 0.1524]   Trim Point: [    0]   Mean LOS: [   3.10]
20 391/15 NORMAL NEWBORN
          Weight: [ 0.1517]   Trim Point: [    0]   Mean LOS: [   3.10]
21 391/15 NORMAL NEWBORN
          Weight: [ 0.1536]   Trim Point: [    0]   Mean LOS: [   3.10]
```

VN stands for "Version" and is the DRG version of the results. The rest of the grouper outputs should be obvious.

Grouper DLL

The Grouper DLL is a programmer's tool.

The DLL is the standard core grouping engine wrapped in a Win32-friendly package. This means that the DLL takes essentially the same input as every other grouping product and gives essentially the same output. Therefore you can use technical information provided about the inputs and outputs of the other grouping products and apply that information to this product.

Sadly, C and BASIC have different function calling conventions. This means that a DLL compiled for C cannot be used by BASIC. Thus all our DLLs come in two flavors. Please be sure that you order the right one.

Choose the VB-Callable DLL (mhdrgvb.dll) to run with Access and Visual BASIC applications.

Choose the C-Callable DLL (mhdrg.dll) to run with applications created with Visual C++ (or some other Win32 C compiler).

Note: as of version 26, released in 2008, the DRG version can have either a 'p' or an 'e' or both appeneded to it. If there is a trailing 'p', it is assumed that the last character of every diagnosis code is a POA flag. If the there is a trailing 'e', then the source institution is presumed to be exempt from the HAC. Thus "26p" specifies POA support, while "26" does not. "25p" does not make sense.

Staying Current

In order to stay up-to-date you have to buy a new one every year.

You get a new masks file with every purchase and the Grouper DLL is backwardly compatible, so if you buy version X one year and version Y the next, you will still be able to assign version X DRGs with the new Grouper DLL.

Technical Details

The Grouper DLL is a Win32 Dynamic Link Library, written in ANSI C and compiled either for use with Visual BASIC software or for use with Visual C++ software.

Distribution

The Grouper DLL is distributed with an installer to allow you to install or uninstall it cleanly.

Calling DLL Functions

Whenever you call a function from a DLL, you must specify the following:

1. the name of DLL file
2. the function prototype, ie what arguments the function takes as input and what result the function gives as output.

The syntax for specifying this information varies from programming language to programming language, but the essential information to be conveyed is the same across all programming languages.

VB Example: DECLARE

In Visual BASIC, the statement you need is the DECLARE statement. Refer to the documentation that came with your VB compiler for details.

Here is a DECLARE statement that worked for us in VB 5:

```
Private Declare Function mhicd Lib "mhicdvb.dll" ( _
    ByVal which As String, _
    ByVal file As String, ByVal code As String, _
    ByVal retval As String, _
    ByVal length As Integer) As Integer
```

All five lines are actually a single statement; the underscores at the end are continuation marks.

Line 1 specifies the DLL (mhicdvb.dll) and the function name (mhicd).

Line 2 specifies that the first argumeent to mhicd() is called "which", is passed by value and is a string.

Line 3 specifies that the second argumeent to mhicd() is called "file", is passed by value and is a string.

Line 4 specifies that the third argumeent to mhicd() is called "retval", is passed by value and is a string.

Line 5 specifies that the fourth argumeent to mhicd() is called "length", is passed by value and is an integer. This line also specifies that mhicd() itself returns an integer value.

C Example: Linking

The ways in which DLLs are exposed to applications varies between different C, or Visual C++, or C# implementations. You will have to consult the documentation for your particular environment for the details of calling out to DLL functions from your software.

We use LCC-Win32 and in this environment, the secret is all in the linking:

```
lc -ansic tryit.c mhdrg.lib mhicd.lib -o tryit.exe
```

Note the references to mhdrg.lib and mhicd.lib; these are stubs which allow the application to call out mhdrg.dll and mhicd.dll respectively.

VB DLL API

The Application Program Interface (API) describes how to call the various functions in the DLL. The API described in this section is the VB-callable DLL or the C-callable DLL.

MHDLLVER

The function mhdllver() is provided to give the programmer access to both the highest support DRG version and the internal versions of the DLL itself and its grouper logic.

```
Dim VerStr As String * 80
Dim MaxVer As Integer

'get the DLL version
MaxVer = mhdllver(VerStr, 79)
```

There are two parameters: a buffer into which to put the version string and a maximum length of that buffer. Note that you have to allocate the memory for the buffer outside the call because this function does not allocate memory for you.

In Visual BASIC, this means using the DIM command with an explicit length.

MHDRG

In-place assignment means that a function takes a point to a variable in the main program and then sets the variable in the main program through that pointer. The alternative is returning a value to the main program.

The function mhdrg() actually assigns the DRG and returns the results. This function does mostly in-place assignment, which is why the DECLARE statement for this function uses the BYVAL keyword.

In order to get around the different ways in which different environments handle binary numbers, most of the parameters are strings even if they represent numbers. Thus patient age is a string, not an integer.

```
ReturnCode = mhdrg(drg,myver,masksdir,_
    mydstat,myage,mysex,mydxbuf,mypxbuf)
```

There are eight parameters:

1. a pointer to an integer into which to put the DRG;
2. a pointer to a string into which to put the DRG version;
3. a pointer to a string into which holds the full path to the directory in which to find the masks files
4. a pointer to a string into which holds the Discharge Status;
5. a pointer to a string which holds the patient age
6. a pointer to a string which holds the patient sex (1=male, 2=female, 0=unknown)
7. a pointer to a string which holds the diagnosis codes, separated by commas
8. a pointer to a string which holds the procedure codes, separated by commas

Note: as of version 26, released in 2008, the DRG version can have either a 'p' or an 'e' or both appeneded to it. If there is a trailing 'p', it is assumed that the last character of every diagnosis code is a POA flag. If the there is a trailing 'e', then the source institution is presumed to be exempt from the HAC. Thus "26p" specifies POA support, while "26" does not. "25p" does not make sense.

Return Code -1

The DLL has a special return code: minus 1 (-1). This code is a generic "initialization failure" code, denoting any of the following conditions:

- missing "sex" parameter
- missing "age" parameter
- missing "version" parameter

- missing "masks path" parameter
- "version" parameter < lowest supported version or > highest supported version

VB Sample Code

What follows is a chunk of Visual BASIC which calls our Grouper DLL:

```
Option Explicit

Private Declare Function mhicd Lib "mhicdvb.dll" ( _
    ByVal which As String, _
    ByVal file As String, ByVal code As String,  _
    ByVal retval As String, _
    ByVal length As Integer) As Integer

Private Declare Function mhdllver Lib "mhdrgvb.dll" ( _
    ByVal Buf As String, _
    ByVal BufLen As Integer) As Integer

Private Declare Function mhdrg Lib "mhdrgvb.dll" ( _
    drg As Integer, _
    ByVal DRGVersion As String, _
    ByVal MasksPath As String, _
    ByVal DischStat As String, _
    ByVal PtAge As String, _
    ByVal PtGender As String, _
    ByVal DXList As String, _
    ByVal ProcList As String) As Integer

Private Declare Sub mherrdesc Lib "mhdrgvb.dll" ( _
    ByVal Buffer As String, _
    ByVal length As Integer)

Private Declare Sub mhinfo Lib "mhdrgvb.dll" ( _
    drg As Integer, _
    ByVal DRGVersion As String, _
    ByVal MasksPath As String, _
    mdc As Integer, _
    weight As Double, _
    los As Double, _
```

```
    ByVal Desc As String, _
    ByVal DescLen As Integer)

Private Declare Function mhcodeused Lib "mhdrgvb.dll" ( _
    ByVal which _
    As String, _
    ByVal codeindex As Integer) As Integer

Private Declare Function mhdrgver Lib "mhdrgvb.dll" ( _
    ByVal MPath As String, _
    ByVal Buf As String, _
    ByVal BufLen As Integer) As Integer

Private Sub AssignDRG()
    Dim ErrMsg As String * 256
    Dim ReturnCode As Integer
    Dim drg As Integer, mdc As Integer
    Dim Desc As String * 80
    Dim weight As Double, los As Double
    Dim masksdir As String
    Dim myver As String,
    Dim mydstat As String,
    Dim myage As String,
    Dim mysex As String
    Dim mydxbuf As String * 80
    Dim mypxbuf As String * 80
    Dim tempStr As String
    Dim N As Integer, needcomma As Integer

    'Loop through controls, getting their current values
    masksdir = Command
    myver = Me!ver
    mydstat = Left$(Me!dstat, 1)
    myage = Me!age
    mysex = Left$(Me!sex, 1)

    'make string out of the diagnoses codes
    tempStr = ""
    needcomma = 0
    For N = 0 To 9
        If Len(Me!dx(N)) > 0 Then
            If needcomma <> 0 Then
                tempStr = tempStr & ","
            End If
```

```
            needcomma = 1
            tempStr = tempStr & Me!dx(N)
        End If
    Next N
    mydxbuf = tempStr

    'make string out of the procedure codes
    tempStr = ""
    needcomma = 0
    For N = 0 To 14
        If Len(Me!proc(N)) > 0 Then
            If needcomma <> 0 Then
                tempStr = tempStr & ","
            End If
            needcomma = 1
            tempStr = tempStr & Me!proc(N)
        End If
    Next N
    mypxbuf = tempStr

    'call the M+H grouper with what you got
    Me!results = ""
    ReturnCode = mhdrg(drg,myver,masksdir,_
        mydstat,myage,mysex,mydxbuf,mypxbuf)

    If ReturnCode <> 0 Then          'drg assignment failed, alas!
        Call mherrdesc(ErrMsg, 70)  'tell user about failure
        Me!results = "DRG Assignment FAILED: " & ErrMsg
    Else                             'drg assignment worked, hurray!
        'get the particulars of this DRG from M+H dll
        Call mhinfo(drg, myver, masksdir, mdc, weight, los, Desc, 80)
        Me!results = "DRG: " & drg & " " & Desc
        Me!info = "MDC: " & mdc & " Weight: " & weight & _
" Mean LOS: " & los & " Version: " & myver

        'which dxes were used?
        For N = 0 To 9
            If mhcodeused("d", N) Then
                Me.dx(N).FontBold = True
            Else
                Me.dx(N).FontBold = False
            End If
        Next N
        'which procs were used?
```

```
        For N = 0 To 14
            If mhcodeused("p", N) Then
                Me.proc(N).FontBold = True
            Else
                Me.proc(N).FontBold = False
            End If
        Next N
    End If

End Sub

Private Sub Form_Load()
    Dim VerStr As String * 80
    Dim MaxVer As Integer
    Dim MPath As String
    Dim DRGVers As String * 81
    Dim N As Integer
    Dim I As Integer

    'expect the masks directory as a command line argument
    If Command = "" Then
        MsgBox (Me.Caption & " " & Chr(10) & Chr(10) & _
        "Required command line argument '" & _
        "Masks Directory' is missing" & _
        Chr(10) & _ "(This is the path to the " & _
        "directory with DRG Masks files and the ICD9 file")
        End
    End If
    MPath = Command

    'get the DLL version
    MaxVer = mhdllver(VerStr, 79)
    Me.Caption = Me.Caption & " " & VerStr

    'get the supported DRG versions
    N = mhdrgver(MPath, DRGVers, 81)     ' deal with error, if any
    I = 1
    Do While N <> 0
        Me.ver.AddItem (Mid$(DRGVers, I, 2))
        If I = 1 Then
            Me.ver.Text = Mid$(DRGVers, I, 2)
        End If
        N = N - 1
        I = I + 2
```

```
    Loop

    'initialize sex list
    Me.sex.AddItem "1 Male"
    Me.sex.AddItem "2 Female"

    'initialize discharge status list
    Me.dstat.AddItem "0 Unknown"
    Me.dstat.AddItem "1 Home"
    Me.dstat.AddItem "2 Other Hosp"
    Me.dstat.AddItem "3 SNF"
    Me.dstat.AddItem "4 ICF"
    Me.dstat.AddItem "5 Other Inst"
    Me.dstat.AddItem "6 Home Care"
    Me.dstat.AddItem "7 AMA"
    Me.dstat.AddItem "8 Expired"
End Sub

Private Sub dx_Change(index As Integer)
    Dim retval As String * 24

    Call mhicd("d", _
        Command & "/icd9.tab", Me.dx(index).Text, retval, 23)
    Me.ddesc(index).Caption = retval
End Sub

Private Sub proc_Change(index As Integer)
    Dim retval As String * 24

    Call mhicd("p", _
        Command & "/icd9.tab", Me.proc(index).Text, retval, 23)
    Me.pdesc(index).Caption = retval
End Sub
```

C Sample Code

What follows is a trivial C program which calls our Grouper DLL:

```
/* tryit.c (c) 2002 M+H Consulting, LLC C-callable demo (BFH) */

#include <stdio.h>
#include <string.h>
```

```
#include <stdlib.h>

#define DELIM "^"

/* DLL functions */
extern int mhicd();             /* mhicd.dll */
extern char * mhdrg();          /* mhdrg.dll */
extern char * mherrdesc();      /* mhdrg.dll */

int main() {
    char * retval;
    char * p;
    char * a[8];
    int i;

#ifdef V23
    /* call the grouper, store results in reval */
    retval = mhdrg(
        "f23",          /* which DRG version you want */
        ".",            /* path to masks files */
        "1",            /* discharge status (home) */
        "34",           /* patient age on discharge */
        "2",            /* patient sex (1=male, 2=female) */
        "V3000",        /* ICD DX codes (single live newborn) */
        "    ",         /* ICD procedure codes (none) */
        5,              /* length of each ICD DX code */
        4               /* length of each ICD procedure code */
    );
#else
    retval = mhdrg(
        "f14",          /* which DRG version you want */
        "d:/mnh/masks", /* path to masks files */
        "8",            /* discharge status (died) */
        "75",           /* patient age on discharge */
        "1",            /* patient sex (1=male, 2=female) */
        /* ICD DX codes */
        "7070 1505 5070 518825990 2859 427891980 1976 1977 ",
        /* ICD procedure codes */
        "8622996099628965939493 96",
        5,              /* length of each ICD DX code */
        4               /* length of each ICD procedure code */
    );
#endif
```

```
    /* if there was an error, alert the user */
    if (retval == NULL) {
        printf("M+H grouper argument or environment error: %s",
        mherrdesc());
        exit(-1);
    }

    /* show the raw return value */
    printf("Raw return value from mhdrg:84s0,retval);

    /* deconstruct return from mhdrg() */
    p = strtok(retval,DELIM);
    for (i = 0; i < 8 && p != NULL; i++) {
        a[i] = p;
        p = strtok(NULL,DELIM);
    }
    puts("Deconstructed return value from mhdrg:");
    printf("rc=%s, mdc=%s, drg=%s, ovn=%s, weight=",a[0],a[1],
        a[2],a[3]);
    printf("%s, mean=%s, porm=%s0esc=%s0,a[4],a[5],a[6],
        a[7]);

    /* while we're at it, check mhicd() */
    if ((i=mhicd("d","icd9.tab","56409",retval))) {
        printf("Error from mhicd(): %d0,i);
    } else {
        printf("%s0,retval);
    }

    return(0);
}

/* This program should produce the following output:
 -------------------------
Raw return value from mhdrg:
0^15^391^20^0.1517^3.10^M^NORMAL NEWBORN

Decontructed return value from mhdrg:
rc=0, mdc=15, drg=391, ovn=20, weight=0.1517, mean=3.10, porm=M
desc=NORMAL NEWBORN
-------------------------
 */
/* eof */
```

IC9cm Name DLL

The ICD9cm Name DLL is a programmer's tool. If you want to include this product as part of software that you sell or lease outside your organization, you will need a Reseller's License. Please refer to Appendix D for details.

Sadly, C and BASIC have different function calling conventions. This means that a DLL compiled for C cannot be used by BASIC. Thus all our DLLs come in two flavors. Please be sure that you order the right one.

Choose the VB-Callable DLL (mhicdvb.dll) to run with Access and Visual BASIC applications.

Choose the C-Callable DLL (mhicd.dll) to run with applications created with Visual C++ (or some other Win32 C compiler).

Staying Current

The structure of our codes table (icd9.tab) stays the same every year, so in order to stay up-to-date you only have to buy a new codes table every year: you can keep using the ICD9 Name DLL that you purchased previously.

Technical Details

The ICD9 Name DLL is a Win32 Dynamic Link Library, written in ANSI C and compiled either for use with Visual BASIC software or for use with Visual C++ software.

Note that the chapter on the Grouper DLL also contains examples of using mhicd.dll and mhicdvb.dll because one often wants to use both of them in the same application.

Distribution

The ICD9 Name DLL is distributed with an installer to allow you to install or uninstall it cleanly.

Calling DLL Functions

Whenever you call a function from a DLL, you must specify the following:

1. the name of DLL file
2. the function prototype, ie what arguments the function takes as input and what result the function gives as output.

The syntax for specifying this information varies from programming language to programming language, but the essential information to be conveyed is the same across all programming languages.

VB Example: DECLARE

In Visual BASIC, the statement you need is the DECLARE statement. Refer to the documentation that came with your VB compiler for details.

Here is a DECLARE statement that worked for us in VB 5:

```
1: Private Declare Function mhicd Lib "mhicdvb.dll" ( _
2:     ByVal which As String, _
3:     ByVal file As String, ByVal code As String,  _
4:     ByVal retval As String, _
5:     ByVal length As Integer) As Integer
```

All five lines are actually a single statement; the underscores at the end are continuation marks.

Line 1 specifies the DLL (mhicdvb.dll) and the function name (mhicd).

Line 2 specifies that the first argumeent to mhicd() is called "which", is passed by value and is a string.

Line 3 specifies that the second argumeent to mhicd() is called "file", is passed by value and is a string.

Line 4 specifies that the third argumeent to mhicd() is called "retval", is passed by value and is a string.

Line 5 specifies that the fourth argumeent to mhicd() is called "length", is passed by value and is an integer. This line also specifies that mhicd() itself returns an integer value.

C Example: Linking

The ways in which DLLs are exposed to applications varies between different C, or Visual C++, or C# implementations. You will have to consult the documentation for your particular environment for the details of calling out to DLL functions from your software.

We use LCC-Win32 and in this environment, the secret is all in the linking:

```
lc -ansic tryit.c mhdrg.lib mhicd.lib -o tryit.exe
```

Note the references to mhdrg.lib and mhicd.lib; these are stubs which allow the application to call out mhdrg.dll and mhicd.dll respectively.

API

The Application Program Interface (API) describes how to call the grouping function in the DLL.

VB Sample Code

What follows is a chunk of Visual BASIC which calls our Grouper DLL:

```
Option Explicit
```

```
Private Declare Function mhicd Lib "mhicdvb.dll" ( _
    ByVal which As String, _
    ByVal file As String, ByVal code As String,  _
    ByVal retval As String, _
    ByVal length As Integer) As Integer

Private Sub dx_Change(index As Integer)
    Dim retval As String * 24

    Call mhicd("d", _
        Command & "/icd9.tab", Me.dx(index).Text, retval, 23)
    Me.ddesc(index).Caption = retval
End Sub

Private Sub proc_Change(index As Integer)
    Dim retval As String * 24

    Call mhicd("p", _
        Command & "/icd9.tab", Me.proc(index).Text, retval, 23)
    Me.pdesc(index).Caption = retval
End Sub
```

C Sample Code

What follows is a trivial C program which calls our ICD9 Name DLL:

```
/* tryit.c (c) 2002 M+H Consulting, LLC C-callable demo (BFH) */

#include <stdio.h>
#include <string.h>
#include <stdlib.h>

#define DELIM "^"

/* DLL functions */
extern int mhicd();             /* mhicd.dll */

int main() {
    char * retval;
    char * p;
```

```
    char * a[8];
    int i;

    /* while we're at it, check mhicd() */
    if ((i=mhicd("d","icd9.tab","56409",retval))) {
        printf("Error from mhicd(): %d0,i);
    } else {
        printf("%s0,retval);
    }

    return(0);
}

/* eof */
```

Perl Shared Object

The Perl shared object is a programmer's tool. If you want to include this product as part of software that you sell or lease outside your organization, you will need a Reseller's License. Please refer to Appendix D for details.

Since the Perl shared object (SO) is a compiled object, it is platform-specific. You have to buy the Perl SO that was compiled for your specific platform. Currently, we only supply the SO under UNIX and UNIX-derived operating systems.

We use an outside porting lab named Ready to Run to provide us with UNIX platforms on which to develop and test, so for an up-to-date list of UNIX variants that we support, please see their web site:

`www.rtr.com`

Note: as of version 26, released in 2008, the DRG version can have either a 'p' or an 'e' or both appeneded to it. If there is a trailing 'p', it is assumed that the last character of every diagnosis code is a POA flag. If the there is a trailing 'e', then the source institution is presumed to be exempt from the HAC. Thus "26p" specifies POA support, while "26" does not. "25p" does not make sense.

Staying Current

In order to stay up-to-date you have to buy a new Perl SO every year.

You get a new masks file with every purchase and the Perl SO is backwardly compatible, so if you buy version X one year and version Y the next, you will still be able to assign version X DRGs with the new Perl SO.

Technical Details

The Perl SO is an interface, written in ANSI C, from which a wrapper was created with SWIG, an open source project to support wrapper generation.

Distribution

The Perl SO is distributed as a file to be installed in the appropriate directory with the appropriate permissions. Since the directory in which the Perl intepreter looks for shared objects varies from installation to installation, we cannot give precise installation instructions.

Calling Perl SO Functions

To call a function in a Perl SO all you have to do is load the SO with the Perl "use" command. Then you can call functions within the SO as if the SO were a Perl package.

Sample Perl Code

What follows is a test program we use to make sure that the Perl SO is working. The package in which the Perl SO is wrapped is called called 'mhdrg'.

The call to mhdrg() should be self-explanatory. You will, of course, have to substitute the correct version number, path to masks files and grouper inputs and output for your installation and your specific data.

mhdrg() takes the usual inputs and gives the usual outputs. For details about how our groupers work, see chapter 2, "DRG Assignment Software." In particular, there is a section on inputs to our grouper and its outputs.

```
# tryit.pl (c) 2002 M+H Consulting, LLC MH DRG test script
use mhdrg;                          # M+H DRG package

# call grouper, store results in $retval
$retval = mhdrg(
```

```
        'f22',                  # which DRG version you want
        '/usr/tmp/drgmasks',    # path to masks files
        '1',                    # discharge status (home)
        '34',                   # patient age on admission
        '2',                    # patient sex (1=male, 2=female)
        'V3000',                # ICD DX codes (single live newborn)
        '    ',                 # ICD procedure codes (none)
        '5',                    # length of each ICD DX code
        '4',                    # length of each ICD procedure code
    );

# if there was an error, alert the user
if ($retval eq '') {
    $msg = "M+H grouper argument or environment error: " .
        mhdrg::errdesc();
    print STDOUT $msg;
    die $msg;
}

# just for prettiness, remove trailing blanks
$retval =~ s/;

# show the raw return value
printf STDOUT ("Raw return value from mhdrg:93s0,$retval);

# deconstruct return from mhdrg()
($rc,$mdc,$drg,$ovn,$weight,$mean,$porm,$desc) = split(//,$retval,-1);
print STDOUT "Deconstructed return value from mhdrg:0;
print STDOUT "rc=$rc, mdc=$mdc, drg=$drg, ovn=$ovn, weight=";
print STDOUT "$weight, mean=$mean, porm=$porm0esc=$desc0;
exit(0);

# This script should produce the following output:
#------------------------
# Raw return value from mhdrg:
# 0^15^391^20^0.1517^3.10^M^NORMAL NEWBORN
#
# Decontructed return value from mhdrg:
# rc=0, mdc=15, drg=391, ovn=20, weight=0.1517, mean=3.10, porm=M
# desc=NORMAL NEWBORN
#------------------------
```

PHP Shared Object

The PHP shared object is a programmer's tool. If you want to include this product as part of software that you sell or lease outside your organization, you will need a Reseller's License. Please refer to Appendix D for details.

Since the PHP shared object (SO) is a compiled object, it is platform-specific. You have to buy the PHP SO that was compiled for your specific platform. Currently, we only supply the SO under UNIX and UNIX-derived operating systems.

We use an outside porting lab named Ready to Run to provide us with UNIX platforms on which to develop and test, so for an up-to-date list of UNIX variants that we support, please see their web site:

`www.rtr.com`

Note: as of version 26, released in 2008, the DRG version can have either a 'p' or an 'e' or both appeneded to it. If there is a trailing 'p', it is assumed that the last character of every diagnosis code is a POA flag. If the there is a trailing 'e', then the source institution is presumed to be exempt from the HAC. Thus "26p" specifies POA support, while "26" does not. "25p" does not make sense.

Staying Current

In order to stay up-to-date you have to buy a new PHP SO every year.

You get a new masks file with every purchase and the PHP SO is backwardly compatible, so if you buy version X one year and version Y the next, you will still be able to assign version X DRGs with the new PHP SO.

Technical Details

The PHP SO is an interface, written in ANSI C, from which a wrapper was created with SWIG, an open source project to support wrapper generation.

Distribution

The PHP SO is distributed as a file to be installed in the appropriate directory with the appropriate permissions. Since the directory in which the PHP intepreter looks for shared objects varies from installation to installation, we cannot give precise installation instructions.

Calling PHP SO Functions

To call a function in a PHP SO all you have to do is load the SO with the PHP "dl" command. Then you can call functions within the SO as if the SO were a PHP package.

In our case, we use the following idiom that we found on the Internet:

```
if (!extension_loaded('mhdrg')) {
    if (!dl('mhdrg.so')) {  // this should be in a protected directory
        exit;
    }
}
```

Sample PHP Code

What follows is a test program we use to make sure that the PHP SO is working. The package in which the PHP SO is wrapped is called called 'mhdrg'.

The call to mhdrg() should be self-explanatory. The rules for calling mhdrg() are the same in Perl or PHP, so we refer you to the chapter on the Perl SO for documentation on the mhcall() itself.

mhdrg() takes the usual inputs and gives the usual outputs. For details about how our groupers work, see chapter 2, "DRG Assignment Software." In particular, there is a section on inputs to our grouper and its outputs.

```
<?php
    # tryit.php (c) 2002 M+H Consulting, LLC MH DRG test script

    if (!extension_loaded('mhdrg')) {
        // this should be in a protected directory
        if (!dl('mhdrg.so')) {
            exit;
        }
    }

    # call grouper, store results in $retval
    $retval = mhdrg(
        'f22',                 # which DRG version you want
        '/usr/tmp/drgmasks',   # path to masks files
        '1',                   # discharge status (home)
        '34',                  # patient age on admission
        '2',                   # patient sex (1=male, 2=female)
        'V3000',               # ICD DX codes (single live newborn)
        '    ',                # ICD procedure codes (none)
        '5',                   # length of each ICD DX code
        '4',                   # length of each ICD procedure code
    );

    # if there was an error, alert the user
    if ($retval == '') {
        $error = errdesc();
        print("Error: $error<br>");
        exit;
    }

    # show the raw return value
    printf("Raw return value from mhdrg:<br>%s<br><br>",$retval);

    # deconstruct return from mhdrg()
    list($rc,$mdc,$drg,$ovn,$weight,$mean,$porm,$desc) =
        explode("^",$retval,-1);
    print("Deconstructed return value from mhdrg:<br>");
    print("rc=$rc, mdc=$mdc, drg=$drg, ovn=$ovn, weight=");
    print("$weight, mean=$mean, porm=$porm<br>desc=$desc<br>");
```

```
    exit;

    # This script should produce the following output:
    #-------------------------
    # Raw return value from mhdrg:
    # 0^15^391^20^0.1517^3.10^M^NORMAL NEWBORN
    #
    # Decontructed return value from mhdrg:
    # rc=0, mdc=15, drg=391, ovn=20, weight=0.1517, mean=3.10, porm=M
    # desc=NORMAL NEWBORN
    #-------------------------
?>
```

C-Callable Object

The C-Callable object is a programmer's tool. If you want to include this product as part of software that you sell or lease outside your organization, you will need a Reseller's License. Please refer to Appendix D for details.

Since the C-Callable object (CO) is a compiled object, it is platform-specific. You have to buy the CO that was compiled for your specific platform. Currently, we only supply the CO under UNIX and UNIX-derived operating systems. For Win32 environments, we provide the Grouper DLL instead.

We use an outside porting lab named Ready to Run to provide us with UNIX platforms on which to develop and test, so for an up-to-date list of UNIX variants that we support, please see their web site:

`www.rtr.com`

Note: as of version 26, released in 2008, the DRG version can have either a 'p' or an 'e' or both appeneded to it. If there is a trailing 'p', it is assumed that the last character of every diagnosis code is a POA flag. If the there is a trailing 'e', then the source institution is presumed to be exempt from the HAC. Thus "26p" specifies POA support, while "26" does not. "25p" does not make sense.

Staying Current

In order to stay up-to-date you have to buy a new CO every year.

You get a new masks file with every purchase and the CO is backwardly compatible, so if you buy version X one year and version Y the next, you will still be able to assign version X DRGs with the new CO.

Technical Details

The CO is written in ANSI C and should link happily into any executable created with any standard UNIX C or C++ or C# compiler.

Distribution

The CO is distributed as a file to be installed in the appropriate directory with the appropriate permissions.

Calling CO Functions

To call a function in a CO all you have to do is link your executable with our CO and presto! you can call functions within the CO as if the CO were a part of your software.

Sample C Code

What follows is a test program we use to make sure that the CO is working.

The call to mhdrg() should be self-explanatory. The rules for calling mhdrg() are the same in Perl or PHP, so we refer you to the chapter on the Perl CO for documentation on the mhcall() itself.

mhdrg() takes the usual inputs and gives the usual outputs. For details about how our groupers work, see chapter 2, "DRG Assignment Software." In particular, there is a section on inputs to our grouper and its outputs.

```
/* tryit.c (c) 2002 M+H Consulting, LLC C-callable demo (BFH) */
/* 10/11/2003 added bit-string of used dx's and used procedures */

#include <stdio.h>
#include <string.h>
#include <stdlib.h>

#define DELIM "^"
#define RETURNED 10
```

```
char * mhdrg();

int main() {
    char * retval;
    char * p;
    char * a[RETURNED];
    int i;
    long mask, dxu, pxu;

    /* call the grouper, store results in reval */
    retval = mhdrg(
        "f22",                  /* which DRG version you want */
        ".",                    /* path to masks files */
        "1",                    /* discharge status (home) */
        "34",                   /* patient age on admission */
        "2",                    /* patient sex (1=male, 2=female) */
        "V3000",                /* ICD DX codes (single live newborn) */
        "    ",                 /* ICD procedure codes (none) */
        5,                      /* length of each ICD DX code */
        4                       /* length of each ICD procedure code */
    );

    /* if there was an error, alert the user */
    if (retval == NULL) {
        printf("M+H grouper argument or environment error: %s",
            errdesc());
        exit(-1);
    }

    /* show the raw return value */
    printf("Raw return value from mhdrg:100s0,retval);

    /* deconstruct return from mhdrg() */
    p = strtok(retval,DELIM);
    for (i = 0; i < RETURNED && p != NULL; i++) {
        a[i] = p;
        p = strtok(NULL,DELIM);
    }

    /* last two return values are bit-strings of which ICD codes were
     * used in the grouping
     */
    dxu = atol(a[8]);
    pxu = atol(a[9]);
```

```
    puts("Deconstructed return value from mhdrg:");
    printf("rc=%s, mdc=%s, drg=%s, ovn=%s, weight=",a[0],a[1],a[2],
        a[3]);
    printf("%s, mean=%s, porm=%s0esc=%s0x flags:%d, px flags: %d0,
        a[4],a[5],a[6],a[7],dxu,pxu);

    /* last two return values are bit-strings of which ICD codes were
     * used in the grouping
     */
    puts("0ignificant ICD codes:");
    for (mask = 1L,i = 0; i < 32; i++, mask *= 2L) {
        if (mask & dxu) {
            printf(" * DX code %2d was used0,(i+1));
        }
    }
    for (mask = 1L,i = 0; i < 32; i++, mask *= 2L) {
        if (mask & pxu) {
            printf(" * Proc code %2d was used0,(i+1));
        }
    }
    exit(0);
}

/* This program should produce the following output:
 ------------------------
Raw return value from mhdrg:
0^15^391^21^0.1536^3.10^M^NORMAL NEWBORN

Deconstructed return value from mhdrg:
rc=0, mdc=15, drg=391, ovn=21, weight=0.1536, mean=3.10, porm=M
desc=NORMAL NEWBORN
dx flags:1, px flags: 0

Significant ICD codes:
 * DX code  1 was used
------------------------
 */
/* eof */
```

Appendix A: The MDCs

This is the list of MDCs as of 2001. They don't change very often, but if you want an up-to-date list, you should consult the office DRG distribution. This list is provided as a convenience and to give you an idea of what MDCs are.

1. Diseases & Disorders of the Nervous System
2. Diseases & Disorders of the Eye
3. Diseases & Disorders of the Ear, Nose, Mouth & Throat
4. Diseases & Disorders of the Respiratory System
5. Diseases & Disorders of the Circulatory System
6. Diseases & Disorders of the Digestive System
7. Diseases & Disorders of the Hepatobiliary System & Pancreas
8. Diseases & Disorders of the Musculoskeletal System & Conn Tissue
9. Diseases & Disorders of the Skin, Subcutaneous Tissue & Breast
10. Endocrine, Nutritional & Metabolic Diseases & Disorders
11. Diseases & Disorders of the Kidney & Urinary Tract
12. Diseases & Disorders of the Male Reproductive System
13. Diseases & Disorders of the Female Reproductive System
14. Pregnancy, Childbirth & the Puerperium
15. Newborns & Other Neonates with Condtn Orig In Perinatal Period
16. Diseases & Disorders of Blood, Blood Forming Organs, Immunolog Disord

17. Myeloproliferative Diseases & Disorders, Poorly Differentiated Neoplasm
18. Infectious & Parasitic Diseases, Systemic or Unspecified Sites
19. Mental Diseases & Disorders
20. Alcohol/drug Use & Alcohol/drug Induced Organic Mental Disorders
21. Injuries, Poisonings & Toxic Effects of Drugs
22. Burns
23. Factors Influencing Hlth Stat & Othr Contacts with Hlth Servcs
24. Multiple Significant Trauma
25. Human Immunodeficiency Virus Infections

Appendix B: Return Codes

The following is a list of valid return codes for DRGGroupers.com groupers, as of 2008. This list is provided to give you an idea of what is returned. Please consult our on-line documentation for an up-to-date list.

`www.drggroupers.com/support.html#T9`

1. means EITHER that there were no diagnosis codes given or that the given principal dx code does not have an MDC (ie is not valid as a principal dx).

2. means no DRG could be found to match MDC and principal dx.

3. means that the given age was not between 0-124.

4. means that the given sex was not 1=male or 2=female

5. is no longer used; Discharge Status is defaulted depending on various factors (disposition status coding system, eg)

6. depends on various factors; for example, for some DRG versions this means that birthweight was not between 200 and 9000 grammes.

7. means that the principal dx code was not a valid choice as a primary diagnosis; the code may be valid, but it is not an allowed starting point for assigning a DRG.

8. means that the DRG masks file could not be found or initialized by the run-time environment.

9. means that the DRG to be labelled is too high for the specified DRG version

10. means that the DRG masks file has internal structural errors.

Appendix C: Discharge Status

The following is a partial list of Discharge Statuses, coded using the UB92 standard. For a more complete list, please see our web site:

`www.drggroupers.com/dstat.pdf`

01 = Home, Self Care

02 = Short Term Hospital

03 = Skilled Nursing Facility

04 = ICF

05 = Other Facility

06 = Home Health Service

07 = Against Medical Advice

08 = Home IV Service

20 = Expired

30 = Still a patient

Appendix D: Software Licenses

There are the standard licenses DRGGroupers.com grants through our parent company, M+H Consulting, LLC.

Reseller License

If you want to embed our grouper in a product you will be selling on the market, then you need to negotiate a custom license agreement. Please contact us for details.

Non-standard Licenses

Our licensing is negotiable and we have granted custom license in past. If you have an arrangement you would like us to consider, contact us.

Contact Information

You can find our up-to-date contact information on-line:

`www.drggroupers.com/contact.html`

Standard Client Software License

M+H Consulting, LLC grants to the purchaser a single CPU license for the accompanying software. The software may not be used on more than one computer at the same time. The purchaser shall not make copies of the software except for use as a backup.

The accompanying software is the property of M+H Consulting, LLC and may not be distributed. The software may not be distributed as part of an application or external website without the express, written consent of M+H Consulting, LLC.

Standard Server Software License

M+H Consulting, LLC grants to the purchaser a single CPU license for the accompanying software. The software may not be used on more than one computer at the same time. The purchaser shall not make copies of the software except for use as a backup.

The software may run on only one CPU, "the server," at a time, but no restriction is placed on how many client CPU's can access the server at a time. However, the purchaser may not put the software on a server to which there is network access outside of the purchaser's organization. In this context, "organization" refers to parent companies and their wholly-owned subsidiaries and business units.

The software is the property of M+H Consulting, LLC and may not be distributed. The program may not be distributed as part of an application or external website without the express, written consent of M+H Consulting, LLC.

Appendix E: File Dictionary

Here is a list of files generated by DRGGroupers.com. This list is provided as a service to our customers, to help you figure out what you have and what you lack in the event of an issue with your installation of any of our offerings.

c32_libmhdrg.so

- Instructions: rename to libmhdrg.so before installing on a 32-bit system

This file is found in the following product:

- 32 bit C-callable shared object (product ID COBJ32SO)

c64_libmhdrg.so

- Instructions: rename to libmhdrg.so before installing on a 64-bit system

This file is found in the following product:

- 64 bit C-callable shared object (product ID COBJ64SO)

cgi-drg.exe

This file is found in the following product:

- 32 bit Windows CGI DRG Assigner (product ID W32CGIDRG)

cgi-drg_32

- Instructions: rename to cgi_drg before installing on a 32-bit system

This file is found in the following product:

- 32 bit Linux CGI DRG Assigner (product ID LINUX32CGIDRG)

cgi-drg_64

- Instructions: rename to cgi_drg before installing on a 64-bit system

This file is found in the following product:

- 64 bit Linux CGI DRG Assigner (product ID LINUX64CGIDRG)

DischargeDispositions.txt

This file is found in the following product:

- MS-Excel DRG Assigning spreadsheet (product ID XLDRG)

drgfilt.aix

- Instructions: rename to drgfilt before installing on an IBM AIX system

This file is found in the following product:

- DRGFilt for AIX (product ID AIXFILT)

drgfilt.exe

This file is found in the following product:

- DRGFilt for 32 bit Windows (product ID WINFILT)

drgfilt.sparc

- Instructions: rename to drgfilt before installing on an Sun SPARC system

This file is found in the following product:

- DRGFilt for Sun SPARC (product ID SPARCFILT)

drgfilt_lnx_32

- Instructions: rename to drgfilt before installing on a 32-bit Linux system

This file is found in the following product:

- 32 bit Linux DRGFilt (product ID LINUXFILT32)

drgfilt_lnx_64

- Instructions: rename to drgfilt before installing on a 64-bit Linux system

This file is found in the following product:

- 64 bit Linux DRGFilt (product ID LINUXFILT64)

drgman.pdf

This file is part of every order. It is our technical documentation as a PDF. This PDF is available for separate purchase in book form from Amazon as well.

icd9.tab

This file is found in the following product:

- ICD9cm short file (product ID ICDTAB)

ide

This file is found in the following product:

- ICL Run-time Environment Upgrade (product ID ICLUP)

mhdrg.exe

This file is found in the following product:

- Visual C-callable DLL (product ID CDLL)

mhdrgvb.exe

This file is found in the following products:

- MS-Excel DRG Assigning spreadsheet (product ID XLDRG)
- VB-callable grouper DLL (product ID VBDLL)

mhdrgvb.xls

This file is found in the following product:

- MS-Excel DRG Assigning spreadsheet (product ID XLDRG)

MHGrouper.mdb

This file is found in the following product:

- MS-Access DRG Assigner (product ID ACCESSDRG)

mhi9tabf26.exe

This file is found in the following product:

- ICD9 Name-finding C-callable DLL (product ID CICD)

mhicdvb.exe

This file is found in the following product:

- ICD9cm Name VB-callable DLL (product ID VBICD)

mhvbdrg.exe

This file is found in the following product:

- Windows desktop app to assign DRGs (product ID VBDRG)

perl32_mhdrg.so

- Instructions: rename to mhdrg.so before installing into a 32-bit Linux Perl path

This file is found in the following product:

- 32 bit Perl-callable shared object (product ID PERL32SO)

perl64_mhdrg.so

- Instructions: rename to mhdrg.so before installing into a 64-bit Linux Perl path

This file is found in the following product:

- Perl-callable shared object (product ID PERL64SO)

php32_mhdrg.so

- Instructions: rename to mhdrg.so before installing into a 32-bit Linux Perl path

This file is found in the following product:

- 32 bit PHP-callable shared object (product ID PHP32SO)

php64_mhdrg.so

- Instructions: rename to mhdrg.so before installing into a 64-bit Linux Perl path

This file is found in the following product:

- 64 bit PHP-callable shared object (product ID PHP64SO)

readme-excel.txt

This file is found in the following product:

- MS-Excel DRG Assigning spreadsheet (product ID XLDRG)

Glossary

The following is a glossary of terms used in this book which may not be familiar to the reader, especially the programmer who is trying to embed a grouper in their software.

The definitions here are not intended to be complete; instead, they are intended to make our descriptions and directions clearer.

Classification

DRGs are classified as either Medical or Surgical because some conditions have both a surgical and non-surgical treatment path and the expected resource consumption of the two paths are quite different.

CPT Codes

The American Medical Association has defined a scheme for coding procedures, which they call CPT (Current Procedural Terminology). For more information, go on-line:

`www.ama-assn.org/ama/pub/category/3113.html`

DRG

DRG stands for Diagnosis Related Group. Inpatient medical records can be classified into separate groups. Each group is identified by a number. This number is the DRG. Each DRG has various attributes associated with it: the description, the Major Diagnostic Category (MDC), the expected Length Of Stay (LOS), the weight (a measure of how resource-intensive it is), a low trim point and a high trim point. See our web site for details:

`www.drggroupers.com/drgs.html`

DRG Grouper

Software that assigns a DRG is called a Grouper. Groupers take coded medical data elements as input and give a DRG as output. The inputs are: age-on-admission, sex, discharge disposition, diagnosis codes (in ICD9cm) and procedure codes (in ICD9cm).

Up to ten diagnoses are considered and the diagnosis codes are assumed to be in order of significance.

Up to fifteen procedures are considered and the procedure codes are assumed to be in order of significance.

DRG Version

A new definition of DRGs is released every October 1st. Each new definition is a new version, requiring a new release of the software and a new masks file.

US Federal (aka CMS or HCFA) DRG versions are released in October of every year. Version 3 (the first version we support) was released in October of 1985. So if you are using calendar years, 1/1/2001 - 9/30/2001 would be covered by version 18 and 10/1/2001 through 9/30/2002 would be covered by version 19. And so on.

The official release is on October 1st every year and we usually release our implementation of the algorithm by October 15th every year.

Please specify which version you need for any of our products. Our module is backwardly compatible, so if you buy the version 10 grouper, that module can handle version 3 through 10, assuming that you have purchased the appropriate masks file.

For our software, version numbers can be preceeded by an optional letter 'f' for federal.

Federal DRGs

The original DRGs were defined by HCFA (now CMS), a part of the United State federal government. We call these DRG definitions "the federal DRGs" For details, see our DRG FAQ on our web site:

`www.drggroupers.com/drgs.html`

HAC (Hospital Acquired Complication)

This is a set of rules which change the DRG assigned for a non-exempt institutation based on any POA flags which are present. This was introduced in US federal DRG assigment with version 26, released in October of 2008.

ICD9cm Codes

The official federal grouper only accepts ICD9cm codes (International Committee on Diseases, version 9, Clinical Modifications) for both diagnoses and procedures. There are two lists of codes: a list of diagnoses and a separate list of procedures. Procedures were originally often called "surgeries". The ICD9cm codes are defined by organ system and have a major and minor component, often written

major.minor

Major Diagnostic Category (MDC)

The MDC is a kind of pre-DRG, a looser category from which the appropriate DRG is chosen. Some analyses are based on this looser category in order to provide a higher-level result. See Appendix A for a listing of MDCs as they were in 2001.

Masks File

The canonical US government grouper, which we call "the federal grouper", applies logic and masks to its input to determine the DRG. The masks are ICD9-specific bit masks representing various conditions. Thus, in order to assign a DRG you need both grouper software, which contains the logic, and the appropriate masks file, which contains the masks.

Our grouper software is 100% backwardly compatible, which means that it can apply the logic of any previous year's version, provided that you have the matching masks file.

We expect masks files to be named

```
drgmasks.fN
```

where N is the version to which they correspond. So the masks file name for version 8 would be

```
drgmasks.f8
```

and the masks file name for version 21 would be

```
drgmasks.f21
```

POA (Present on Admission)

In order to avoid paying for medical mistakes, diagnoses are now flagged as having been present on admission (POA).

The values for the POA flag are not, as one might expect, simply Y or N; rather the following options are defined:

- Y for Yes -N for No -U for Unspecified -W for clinically undetermined -1 for unreported / not used / exempt from reporting

Return Code

Our groupers always return a code which indicate success (a value of zero) or some kind of failure (a non-zero value). For details on the possible kinds of failure, you can refer to the list in Appendix B, or our tech support page on our web site:

Significant Code Bit String (dflg and sflg)

Not all the codes, either diagnosis or procedure, are significant in determining the DRG. Our groupers will tell you which codes were used in the DRG assignement and which were not.

This information is conveyed by a string of either ones or zeros. For historical reasons, this string of characters is referred to as "the bit string."

There are ten input Diagnosis codes, and so there are ten digits in the Diagnosis bit string. There are fifteen input Procedure codes, so there are fifteen digits in the Procedure bit string.

If a given digit is zero, then the corresponding code was not used; if a given digit is one, then the corresponding code was used.

`www.drggroupers.com/support.html#T10`

Index